Epigenetics and the Psychology of Weight Loss

How to Lose More Weight with Less Effort

Dr. Francisco M. Torres, MD

Contents

Disclaimer

This book is to be used for educational purposes only. It should not be used to treat, diagnose, prescribe, or substitute for personal medical advice.

Consult a medical professional before starting or trying any new substance, treatment, or exercise regimen.

Likewise, any ingredient, herbal or otherwise, should always be reviewed for safety, as well as contraindications with any current medications in consultation with your qualified healthcare provider.

Neither the author nor the publisher accepts any responsibility for the actions of readers of this book.

For Dr. Gerty Jones. You showed me what it means to go above and beyond, and inspired me to get moving.

PREFACE

It is seldom that we as human beings get the opportunity to reflect on and comprehend the inner workings of our intrinsic value and what that value means in the brief ripple that represents our individual lifetime.

Identifying what that value is starts with fostering a deeper and more intentional understanding of what makes us tick and why we make decisions the way we do. In a very simple yet complex sense, the way in which we choose to view ourselves, the importance of our health, the value we carry of others in relationships, and the way in which we manage life's constant stressors all have a direct impact on how we identify the value we carry as human beings.

In the pages that follow, I warmly invite you to give yourself permission to grow and embody the wisdom my esteemed colleague Dr. Francisco Torres provides. His deep and thorough analysis of individual psychology coupled with a clear and concise explanation of how surroundings influence your biology are uniquely fused with applicable and easy steps to take greater control of yourself so you can live your absolute best life.

We live in a modern age of "connected disconnection"; we are more connected to each other than ever through technology, yet incredibly disconnected in the understanding we have of ourselves and our "why." Most diet and self-help books across the country do a really good job at giving you a basic "to-do" blueprint but often fall short when it comes to improving your own understanding of why you choose to engage in certain behaviors, crave particular foods, and choose a lifestyle that is not conducive to your optimal well-being.

A focal point in this masterpiece by Dr. Torres is the focus, elaboration, and explanation of stress as well as anxiety and how they directly contribute to chronic pain, unhealthy weight gain, acceleration of aging, and the very real necessity of slaying dragons that fuel detrimental behaviors and could be passed onto your children.

The pages that follow are priceless, literally. If adhered to and followed they have the very real potential of positively changing your life and the life of those you love.

Nothing is more valuable in this world than time. What separates us as human beings is what we do with that time and how it influences those we have the privilege to love and share life with.

Like you, I want to have a lasting impact and make the brief ripple that is my existence truly mean something special to myself and those around me. That starts with having a deeper understanding of my own psychology, biology, and environment to ensure I have the right ingredients to live a healthy, happy, and vibrant life; Dr. Torres provides that exact roadmap to achieve this in the pages that follow.

Enjoy the journey and embody the wisdom provided to you by Francisco; I have, and it has made a tremendous difference in my life and the life of those I love.

Dr. Gino Collura
    Author of *Seven Layers of Successful Relationships*
    Behavioral Scientist and National Speaker

INTRODUCTION

If you have read my memoir, *Keep Kicking Frisco, Keep Kicking*, you know I have struggled with weight and body image issues throughout my life. My early childhood was characterized by profound shame over my appearance and a crippling anxiety that turned out to be primarily related to epigenetic "switches" in my DNA. Thankfully, as this book discusses, switches can be flipped to "off."

As of the last decade, I thought I had overcome my physical challenges once and for all. I lost weight, got fit, and even did well in amateur bodybuilding competitions. I got my panic attacks under control, and I felt better than ever. My medical practice expanded to help patients follow in my footsteps. Many of my clients were successfully achieving the bodies of their dreams and lifting the weight of anxiety from their lives. As far as I was concerned, I had made it.

Then the COVID-19 pandemic happened.

A global health emergency of this baffling, highly contagious, and often fatal virus was not a good thing for me as a medical doctor with an anxiety disorder. As hospitals overflowed and talk of a global supply chain collapse became part of our daily news cycle, my anxiety spiked.

To top it all off, my exercise routine fell apart. I no longer had as much reason to walk in my daily life. Attending gyms and group fitness classes was no longer safe. I tried to exercise at home, but the combination of anxiety and a sedentary lifestyle proved fateful. After going weeks without exercising, I tried to jump back into my old, aggressive workout routine. Instead of getting fit, I ended up severely injuring my knee and rendering myself *unable* to exercise for weeks.

So, yes. I gained my "COVID 19" (19 pounds, that is) during 2020, as a result of my anxiety and newly sedentary lifestyle. To make matters worse, I found myself unable to get back on my exercise program, even if I wanted to. My doctors said I would be unable to begin exercising again until I underwent major surgery to repair several components of my torn knee.

In the space of just a few months, I felt as though I had lost several years' worth of progress. Then a new monster began to creep in: doubt.

Was I qualified to teach patients to lose weight and stay healthy and fit if I could not even do it myself? Didn't my weight gain prove that I was a fraud? Did my injury suggest that my exercise program did not work to keep people healthy as well as I had advertised?

We all struggle and have setbacks in our journeys to health and fitness. As the pandemic proceeded, I saw many of my patients fall into the same despair. How could they stay healthy and fit under the stress of a global pandemic? How could they keep exercising if they had no reason to leave their house? Did the relapses they were having right now mean that they too were frauds, and that their health and weight loss journeys were doomed to fail?

Seeing my patients struggle with these fears made me realize I needed to do something. We all struggle with setbacks, with or without a global pandemic: they are part of the journey. With so many people struggling, I decided I needed to do something to help.

The best thing I could do, the most valuable and honest, would be to rehabilitate myself first.

This time, I started slowly. I was gentle with myself. Nevertheless, I was persistent. I had a mission. I would show my patients that we could all come back from the chaos that was 2020 and that a setback did not mean defeat.

I began eating healthy again. I began exercising gently and mindfully, putting my clinical knowledge to full use. Soon, my doctors were astonished to see that I had done the impossible: I had regained full range of motion in my knee and was able to do weight-bearing exercises without pain, even though my MRI had shown multiple injuries, which *should* have required surgery to repair.

I had also lost weight—enough that I resolved to return to the amateur bodybuilding competition circuit in the fall of 2021, just to prove that I could.

As of today, I am registered for my first Masters' Physique bodybuilding competition in years. I am back to a full range of athletic capabilities. Moreover, I look and feel great.

Do you know what that means?

It means you can do it, too.

I started with many genetic disadvantages in life. As an overweight child and a teen suffering from a panic disorder, I was not someone people might someday have expected to become a bodybuilder or a thrill-seeker. Beneath my apparent struggles, my DNA was deeply programmed with generations of trauma dating to the Spanish Civil War and earlier. My parents also suffered from psychiatric illnesses due in part to this inherited trauma, which explained many of our familial health problems.

However, the past is not the whole story. The future is ours to write.

This book focuses on two primary research areas to help us make long-term changes for ourselves—and maybe even for future generations of our families. These are:

1. **Psychology**. We will learn to adopt thinking patterns that make it easier for us to reach all of our goals, no matter how difficult they may seem at first.
2. **Epigenetics**. We will explore how the expression of our DNA can be altered by our lifestyle choices, including diet, exercise, and choices we make that may affect our mood. This is particularly remarkable because these epigenetic changes may be passed on to any children we have after making these changes to our cells.

In this book we will discuss a healthy diet, powerful exercise, and the science of epigenetics. We will discuss how familial and personal trauma can alter our DNA, making us more prone to obesity and other diseases, and how to change our DNA *back*, healing personal and generational trauma for future generations with the right lifestyle choices.

To help you meet your priorities as fast as possible, the contents of this book are broken down by specific goals. Remember that every goal we discuss in this book is part of the same system which is designed to help us survive. For that reason, use what you learn in *all* the chapters to achieve optimal epigenetic effects. Every lifestyle change recommended in this book supports every goal in this book, directly or indirectly.

The goals we will focus on include:

1. Weight loss.
2. Reducing chronic pain.
3. Slowing the aging process.
4. Passing on healthier habits and genetic memories to the next generation.

This book is unique. It is not only about making practical lifestyle changes. And it is not only about the academic science of epigenetics. I have written this book to include both aspects, ensuring that you know *why* these lifestyle changes work, and what the practical importance of these scientific discoveries is to your life.

I am passionate about losing weight naturally, not by using artificial and potentially unhealthy diet aids or surgeries. In life, it is the journey that matters and the series of skills you gain along the way. The destination is only part of the real goal.

I am eager to share this book with you. I know that you will find as much success in your journey as I have found in mine. And I wish you even more.

Chapter 1

Activate Your Genes, Change Your Life

We all want to feel good and look good. As a doctor, I prioritize feeling good over looking good, but it is a happy accident that many of the same lifestyle changes which result in weight loss also result in improved health. Throughout this book, we will explore lifestyle changes that can result in improved health and longevity, with weight loss as a happy side effect along the way. We will also examine what psychological science teaches us about how to actually *make* these lifestyle changes and make them stick.

Wrapped up in all this is the budding field of epigenetics. This astonishing field of study shows that, even if we can't change what genes we inherit, we *can* change our gene expression, turning genes on and off within our bodies. Astonishingly, we can even pass these epigenetic changes along to future generations!

Scientists have long understood that our genes determine a great deal about our appearance, our health, and even our emotions and behavior. For many years, the assumption was that the genes we are born with cannot be changed and therefore the hand we are dealt in the cosmic game of genetic poker determines our fate to a large extent. For decades it was believed that some people were simply genetically luckier than others, and people who were born a certain way likely could not change.

This old idea turns out not to be true.

Our genes do contain our "source code," a kind of genetic operating system with instructions for every single task our cells "know" how to do. At its most basic level this source code cannot be changed through natural means. As of this writing, gene therapies are being developed to add and delete bits of our cells' source code, but these are only available for specific, acute medical conditions, so we will leave these out of our discussion.

However, it turns out there is another layer of natural programming written *on top* of our unchangeable genes. This programming allows our cells to adapt to our external circumstances, which, as we all know, can vary wildly. Our programming *can* be changed by our activities, choices, experiences, and life events. When we understand how to use this programming layer, we can turn specific genes on, off, up, or down.

This is an astonishing discovery! It shows us that our choices have far more power to transform our lives—and even the life experiences of future generations of our families—than was once believed. Acts ranging from eating choices to engaging in physical exercise or psychotherapy can change our cells' biochemical programming and how our "source code" is expressed.

This book will delve into the power and function of epigenetics. I will include simple explanations of the biochemistry and laboratory evidence that teach us how to change the activation patterns of our DNA and explain why these methods work. Know that the science contained here is credible and supported by current research.

Before we begin talking about taking control of our lives, let us start with some basic concepts in genetics and biochemistry.

INHERITING OUR SOURCE CODE

Scientists have long known that living things tend to "take after" their ancestors. For centuries, scientists debated how and why people, plants, and animals inherited traits from one parent or another (or even a grandparent or great-grandparent). By "traits," we mean characteristics ranging from hair color and facial features to behaviors, emotions, and eating habits.

In the 19th century, monk and scientist Gregor Mendel became the first person in modern history to study trait inheritance systematically. He concluded traits were passed down from one generation to the next and that some traits, called recessive traits, could even skip generations and show up in grandchildren or great-grandchildren. However, he did not know how any of these traits were transmitted. Was it some mystical intelligence that told the body how to develop? Was it some chemical substance contained in the sperm and the uterus that contained these instructions for new life?[1]

In the 20th century, a new generation of scientists understood how our traits are passed down to us from our parents. It was found that any time a living cell divided, both of its offspring received equal amounts of a chemical substance called DNA. Cells always doubled their amount of DNA—possibly "copying" their stores of this chemical substance—before dividing to make a new cell. Could DNA be the seat of the information that makes us ourselves? If so, how did that work?

In 1953, James Watson and Francis Crick used radiographic images created by Rosalind Franklin to make a breakthrough discovery by identifying the helical structure of DNA. Watson and Crick realized DNA was composed of two different chemical strands twined together—a double helix.[2]

This paved the way for a scientific revolution in genetic studies. The two strands of the helix showed how DNA could be copied and passed on to the next generation. Later scientists discovered that, before a cell divides, the two strands "unzip" from each other. The cell then builds a new DNA strand, using each old DNA strand as a template. This is possible because chemical bonding rules instruct the cell's enzymes precisely how to copy information from one DNA strand to create a new strand.

The result? Each cell has two full copies of its DNA source code when this process is complete. It can then divide in two, bequeathing one copy of these vital instructions to each daughter cell. This is how all living organisms grow and reproduce. When two parents have a child, the child receives half of their DNA from each parent. Egg and sperm cells have clever ways of "remixing" DNA, ensuring that each child receives a unique combination of genes from each parent.

All talented engineers know that redundancy is safe, and nature knows it too. For this reason, animals like humans are "diploid"—"di," meaning "two" and "ploid" meaning "form."[3] This means that each cell receives two copies of every gene we have. This ingenious redundancy means that our bodies have *two* versions of every gene. If one version is damaged we have a backup, and we can even have two versions of the same gene with different, complementary strengths.

In fact, we now know that genetic diversity is essential to population survival because it ensures that each population has many different versions of each gene, and each version is ready to respond to different survival challenges. Genetic diversity ensures that our children have many combinations of behaviors, disease resistance, health traits, and personality traits. This diversity turns out to be necessary because the more genetically diverse a population—that is, the more versions of each gene that can be found within the population—the higher the chance that at least *some* members of the population will be prepared to cope with any adversity that comes.[4]

The fundamental unit of genetic information within living systems is termed a "gene." A gene is an instruction for a single protein or a single chemical building block within a cell. Most life functions require *many* proteins to function and are influenced by many genes.[5]

DNA does not manage itself, however. Instead, it serves as a chemical blueprint to make the components that run our cells. To "express" or "use" a gene, a protein called a transcription enzyme creates a copy of DNA out of a similar but slightly different chemical called RNA. The RNA code may then be changed by other proteins, depending on the instructions it contains.

Once all changes have been made, this RNA is referred to as "mRNA," with the "m" standing for "messenger." The final, edited snippet of instruction, called mRNA, is then "read" by cellular machinery made of more RNA and proteins. This machinery "reads" the instructions and uses them to put together the correct amino acids in the proper order to create a protein.

Think of mRNA as the paper message that is actually delivered to the assembly line workers, telling them how to make the parts our cells need to survive. Because it is only a copy, changes to mRNA may be made safely without risking damage to the master blueprint. [6] The same master DNA blueprint may even be used to make different parts—different proteins—if different alterations are made to the mRNA copies.

Coincidentally, this is also why mRNA vaccines like the vaccine used to teach our immune system to fight COVID cannot change our DNA. Messenger RNA molecules are just disposable copies of information which are used briefly to make cellular parts. Then the mRNA is broken down by enzymes so that our cells don't make too many of these parts. One major challenge for scientists designing mRNA vaccines was actually making the mRNA last long enough inside our cells to be useful!

If this process sounds very complex, it is. Its very power lies in that complexity. At every stage of transcribing DNA into protein, there is the potential for the body to make "choices." A given gene can be used more or less often. One version of the gene may be used, or a different version may be used. This can result in our cells having different component parts, or different amounts of certain component parts. Our cells can actually change at the molecular level as a result of these choices.

So how can we influence the expression of our genes with our own day-to-day lifestyle choices?

CHANGING OUR CELLULAR PROGRAMMING

The process by which our gene expression is modified is called "epigenetics"— "epi" meaning "on top of, above, or besides," and "genetics" referring to the heritable "source code" written in our DNA. Epigenetic instructions can literally be "on top" of our genetic blueprints, often consisting of layers of chemicals that are laid down on top of our DNA by enzymes in order to change how our genetic blueprint is expressed.

Epigenetic instructions can encourage or discourage cells from using any gene, or even change the processing of a gene after it is copied into RNA. In this way they can change the chemical building blocks our cells make, and the biochemical ways in which our cells perform their life functions. This allows our cells to adapt to many external circumstances.

Once we understand how our cells "read" signals from the outside world and use them to "decide" which genes to express and which building blocks to create, we can learn how to gain some control over this process. That's what this book is all about.

There are limits to how much epigenetics can change our gene expression. Unfortunately, if we have a genetic disease where our cells have no working copy of a gene, epigenetic modifications cannot create one. Similarly, epigenetics cannot entirely delete a harmful gene. However, epigenetics can encourage the expression of desired genes while turning "down" the expression of undesired genes.[7] This can change our brain function, weight and fat storage, blood sugar, blood pressure, and more.

Here, we will focus on lifestyle choices to accomplish several specific health and wellness goals. These goals are intimately related at the biochemical level and achieving each one will make you better at the others. Our bodies are holistic systems: the same stress responses that create anxiety and pain sensitivity also encourage our bodies to store fat and speed up aging.

These responses exist for a reason—when being chased by a lion, for example, it is good to have high blood sugar and high blood pressure to keep your cells fueled with plenty of food and oxygen while running. If you get a chance to take a break while being chased, it is a good idea to eat as many high-energy carbs and store as much high-energy fat as possible to continue fueling your cells. If these changes speed up the aging process or make us feel not so great, so be it: that is better than running out of blood sugar to fuel our muscles and being eaten by a lion.

The problem in the modern world is that these stress responses are often triggered when we do not need them. Getting an email from your boss may trigger the same fight-or-flight response as getting chased by a lion, but high blood sugar and feeling anxious will not help you in this situation.[8] The sight of a tasty donut while you are stressed may trigger a belief that you need that donut to survive, but in reality, you probably don't.

These responses, too, can be turned "up" or "down" epigenetically. As we will soon see, people with individual or even family histories of trauma often have their stress responses turned "up" as a remnant of needing to survive times of danger and deprivation. People with such epigenetic "memories" stored in their cells are more likely to experience stress responses like anxiety, depression, fat gain, unhealthy food cravings, and the corresponding more rapid aging that comes from the body's systems being in overdrive.

Even if we do not *know* that our parents or grandparents experienced famine or war, our cells may still "remember" through passed-on epigenetic changes that turn "up" these stress responses. These responses once helped us survive in a world where we really may have been at risk of going hungry or having to outrun an attacker.[9]

However, we *can turn off these responses*. By sending our cells the proper chemical signals through diet, exercise, and psychotherapy, we can switch our genes into the modes of relaxation, optimum health, and longevity. We can chemically "tell" our bodies that there is no lion and no famine; our cells do not need to raise blood sugar, or store fat, or make us worry about every little thing.

Instead, we can relax. And then we can thrive. We can live long, healthy lives. We can even pass on these habits, and these genetic changes, to future generations of our families.

I want to share a story with you now of a truly powerful transformation I have had the privilege of witnessing. If any story illustrates how we are not limited by our genes or our past, it is the story of my patient, Jim.

Chapter 2

Obesity, Pain, and Transformation

When my patient Jim first walked into my clinic, I believed he was going to die. He had already received the most powerful surgical and pharmaceutical interventions available to him, and he was still morbidly obese and in excruciating pain. His obesity and pain were so severe that they were endangering his life, and causing doctors to refuse him more drugs or surgery for fear that these would kill him. Jim was sent to me as a last resort, and at first it seemed to me that Jim was not long for this world.

Today, Jim is one of the most remarkable success stories I have seen or read about in medicine. He is a healthy, fit, active 74-year-old who works out at home daily, eats a healthy diet, and is considering taking up again the more adventurous and athletic hobbies from his youth. He has defied multiple medical diagnoses and well outlived the previous generations of his family.

How did Jim accomplish this? That's what this book is all about. In this chapter, we will see Jim's own account of what has enabled him to transform and grow. Jim's experiences closely match my own recommendations as both a pain management and age management physician. He describes both the psychological and physical journey he undertook to obtain superior results for himself. Throughout the rest of this book, we will look in more detail at the science behind the changes which allowed Jim to heal himself.

For me and Jim, losing weight was a matter of improving our health and our quality of life, not our appearance. The same diet which gave me an unflattering paunch was also contributing to my anxiety. The same lack of exercise was also inflicting back pain and made me vulnerable to serious injury.

For me, the cosmetic rewards were motivating—but weight loss occurred at least in part as a side effect of getting healthier. The same is true for many people. While research is not clear about when and how health problems are caused by obesity, there is reason to suspect that for some, obesity makes it harder to stay healthy.

I want to emphasize uncertainty about the role of obesity in certain health conditions because serious conditions are missed in overweight patients with alarming frequency. Stories abound of doctors finding cancers or dangerous infectious diseases in overweight patients that previous doctors had neglected to even test for because they assumed all of a patients' symptoms were caused solely by their weight.

This failure of due diligence by doctors is likely one of the major contributors to poorer health outcomes among overweight people. The problem is not *just* that excess fat can cause some health conditions; it is also that doctors can under-diagnose and under-treat dangerous conditions in overweight patients due to erroneous assumptions that all of the patient's symptoms are caused strictly by their weight.

That being said, there does come a point where excess weight can take a serious toll on someone's joints, mobility, and cardiovascular function. In cases where excess weight makes exercise difficult or impossible or exacerbates pre-existing issues, this excess weight can result in poor quality of life and a shortened lifespan.

Jim was such a patient.

Jim turned his life around—including both his health and his BMI —with the help of diet and exercise. He came to me as a patient with poor quality of life and a grim prognosis, suffering from extreme chronic pain which had exceeded the capacity of opioid medication to safely treat. His mobility was impaired to the point that he had had to sell his business and was essentially bedridden.

Looking at Jim today, you might imagine that he has been a healthy, active athlete his whole life. You might wrongly assume that a lifestyle like Jim's is out of reach for you because you suffer from challenges with weight, chronic pain, injuries, or lack of confidence around exercise. But this story will prove that none of these things will hold you back.

Jim started with the deck stacked against him in almost every possible way. But his persistence, determination, and the help of a few caring professionals have allowed him to achieve a lifestyle that many 70-somethings may feel is unattainable for them.

We will explore Jim's journey from a 50-something 400-pound man who was almost bedridden with chronic pain to a 70-something healthy 200-pound man with a zest for life and a fitness routine that many 20-somethings could aspire to replicate. In the latter part of his journey, Jim has even used exercise and physical therapy to fight age-related conditions which his doctors told him were untreatable.

Jim's story is proof that transformation through diet and exercise is possible for anyone, regardless of what health challenges you face or how out-of-shape you may feel. Every single person can enjoy drastically improved health and wellness by using diet and exercise, and the understanding that the information we put into our bodies in the form of food, activity, and stressful or enriching stimuli determine the gene expression that our cells put out.

JIM'S STORY

When I first saw Jim as a patient, he was in agonizing pain. His prognosis did not look good. A back injury had forced him to stop working and sell his beloved business. He was now taking as many opiates as he safely could to manage his pain, and it still wasn't enough.

He also weighed 400 pounds. And this was *after* having bariatric surgery to attempt to reduce his weight. Obviously, this severely limited his mobility and put more stress on his injured back. It also put pressure on his lungs and airway, further concerning doctors who worried about the suppression of his breathing–the leading cause of death from opiate overdose.

Jim's doctors had first recommended him for spinal surgery to try to improve his back pain. The surgeons sent him to me because they were afraid that, due to his weight and the pressure on his lungs and throat, he would die under anesthesia. I was tasked specifically with giving Jim spinal injections for his pain. The hope was to find any stopgap treatment that might ease his pain enough to allow some weight loss or reduction in his growing need for opiate treatment. I was determined to help him in any way I could.

Unfortunately, I was not optimistic. His size made it difficult for me to even administer his injections safely. To do so, I needed to find the outline of his bones, which is necessary to safely deliver an injection into the spine without damaging spinal nerve tissue. This was almost impossible to do with Jim's excess body fat.

This guy is gonna die, I thought as I watched Jim wince with pain while my hands felt for his spinal bones. He was a classic grim profile: his pain and his obesity would each work to make the other difficult to heal. Exercise to lose weight would be almost impossible with his level of pain, and his weight would put pressure on his injury and make exercise to strengthen his injured muscles painful and dangerous. Doctors do not expect good prognoses when they see patients in these situations.

Still, I was determined to do all I could for Jim. Maybe, just maybe, he would be the patient who defied the odds.

Fortunately, I learned that Jim shared my optimism. Although life had dealt him many traumas and it seemed that modern medicine had failed him so far, he was not ready to give up. Instead, he was receptive when I talked about lifestyle changes that could improve his condition slowly over time.

Despite all the challenges Jim faced, he was willing to believe that changing his eating and his exercising habits might help his pain.

From my perspective, my own role in Jim's turnaround has been small. I lent a sympathetic ear, and I shared with him my own story of moving from a place of lifelong weight struggles and body image issues to competing in ultramarathons and bodybuilding competitions. I have given diet and exercise advice, and reassurance, where I can. To me, this is what any good doctor should do. I hesitate to take any credit for Jim's progress, because without his own persistence my advice would have been useless.

However, while working on this book, Jim and my editor have both insisted that I share here the things I did that Jim feels helped him to succeed. In our interviews about his success, Jim was emphatic that my care, and the care and skill of other health and exercise professionals, has been integral to his transformation. Hopefully these accounts can serve as a guide for others who want to support colleagues, patients, and loved ones in their health journeys.

Jim is a big fan of my books. Not this one, obviously, since it wasn't available when we first met. But I am also the author of a series of books about diet, exercise, and my own story, *Keep Kicking, Frisco*, which people tell me is at least very entertaining. I have done my best to share my own knowledge and experience with weight loss, exercise, and changing my relationship with food as someone who grew up with an overweight and un-athletic self-image.

Such journeys involve both practical knowledge of nutrition and exercise, and spiritual knowledge of one's worth and one's place in the world. I have done my best to give readers of my books a journey to follow along which incorporates both sides of this coin.

In our interview, Jim went so far as to assert that my other books should be required reading because of their combination of compassion with a no-nonsense approach. I don't know about that myself, but I'll pass the recommendation along on behalf of someone who has been extremely successful in weight loss and healing from chronic pain.

According to Jim, the level of support he got from me as a health-care provider was also important to his success. He insisted I tell you about the time that his daughter called me in a panic after Jim, suffering from symptoms of COVID, was turned away from an Emergency Room.

In the early days of the pandemic, this ER was not sure how to handle the influx of critically ill and highly contagious patients they were receiving. Jim himself was not critically ill, so he was turned away; but he *was* in a high-risk group for severe illness for several reasons, and at this time it was not clear just how inevitable severe illness was for high-risk patients.

Because of the bias whereby mild illness went undiagnosed in some patients, severe COVID was being over-reported, and at the time it looked as though the mortality risk for patients in Jim's age and weight group who contracted COVID could be over 10%.

Upon receiving a series of frantic calls from Jim's daughter, I called her back and asked her for more details about her father's situation. Fortunately, I was able to ascertain that he was not at death's door and could safely return home and monitor his symptoms for signs of severe illness.

After reassuring Jim's daughter that her father sounded like he was likely safe to care for himself at home, I called Jim to learn more. I then called his daughter back to further reassure her that I had spoken with her father and did not consider his case to be dangerous at the moment.

Now, to me, this is doctoring 101. When you have a responsibility to your patients, you must take their concerns seriously and apply your medical knowledge however you can to help them. The fact that it was a Friday after business hours did not even occur to me. But to Jim and his family, my attention and care was so remarkable that they felt the need to bring it up years later, and to ensure that I understood how beneficial my attitude had been to his medical course.

You may question what this anecdote has to do with Jim's weight loss. Well, it is simply this: patients are more likely to follow a doctors' advice diligently when they feel that the doctor truly cares for them. The difference between feeling lectured and judged—a negative and unhelpful experience which does not inspire confidence in a doctor's advice—and feeling supported and cared for is a matter of warm attention.

Does the doctor or other professional helper seem irritated with the patient, as though the patient's health and noncompliance is an inconvenience for the practitioner? Or do they seem concerned because they fear that the patient will come to harm? Patients are much more likely to follow medical advice when they sense that it is being given out of genuine concern for their positive outcome, and not to simply lighten the practitioners' workload or force the patient to conform to some externally enforced ideal.

By answering Jim's after-hours calls and going out of my way to make sure everyone in the family was comfortable and informed, I had demonstrated genuine concern for my patient in all aspects of his life.

To me this did not seem an extraordinary feat, but unfortunately, I hear from too many patients that they have struggled to find doctors who seem warm and invested in their health. When doctors come across as cold and judgmental, that does not make it easier for patients to trust or follow their advice.

Perhaps herein lies a simple, easily replicable tip for doctors and other health practitioners: caring for patients counts. Although so many of us are overwhelmed with hospitals and healthcare practices pressuring us to see dozens of patients per day, patients can tell when we feel we don't have time for them. They can tell when we are impatient or frustrated. They can also tell when we really care about them and are delivering advice out of a genuine belief that better outcomes are possible.

This care and belief costs little to administer. It is available to doctors operating in every healthcare system in the world. So let us never forget the importance of "soft" variables in patient outcomes. If I had delivered care with an attitude of impatience or frustration, Jim tells me, his journey may not have turned out the same.

In time trust grew up between us. Upon first seeing me, Jim had already endured the gauntlet of many doctors who prescribed unsuccessful or unsustainable treatment. He had probably had some doctors who expressed disappointment in his outcomes or the belief that he was failing to follow doctors' orders. He probably expected me to judge him negatively and blame him for the failure of these previous treatment approaches.

And he was sent to me strictly for pain relief. I was not his primary care provider: I was just the guy with the needle who could inject cortisone into his spine.

But as we got to know each other, our appreciation for each other grew. I realized that Jim was a hard worker and a dedicated family man. A doctor glancing at him for the first time, seeing the weight he maintained after bariatric surgery, may have incorrectly attributed his obesity to carelessness rather than to an anxious sense of scarcity that came from having to work for every penny he ever made, or an excessive degree of workaholism which led Jim to put his own health and fitness last behind providing for his family and his employees.

As I opened my eyes to Jim, he began to connect with me in ways he did not connect with other doctors. He felt that I not only cared about his well-being, but that I was willing to share challenging and personal thoughts with him that went beyond the clinical distance of other doctors he'd experienced. According to Jim, I did not merely treat him as a patient: I treated him as a fellow human being whose struggles I was familiar with from my own life.

In time, Jim felt comfortable sharing with me about his personal life. He had a son whose mental illness challenges were a source of great anxiety for Jim and his wife, contributing to his comforting himself with large doses of food. After years of severe pain and obesity he did not see himself as someone who could exercise or diet successfully. But when I spoke about my own exercise and diet practices, he showed interest.

That spark of interest, to a doctor, is worth a patient's weight in gold. In a somewhat literal sense: the more overweight a patient, the more we treasure seeing that spark of initiative. We cannot *make* our patients do anything for their own health, after all, and often we assume that unsolicited recommendations about diet and exercise will not be followed. But when a patient shows an active interest, asks questions, and looks like they think they can really do it, it makes our day. I decided to do whatever I could to encourage Jim's interest.

As it became clear that Jim was serious about exercising, in his words, I "took off my doctor's hat and put on my coach's hat." Wellness coaching was something I'd always been passionate about, exercising that passion through my Forever Young MD business.

Even though Jim was a patient of my pain management practice, not a weight loss or age management patient, I was happy to pursue the same results for him. In Jim's case, his obesity appeared to be exacerbating his pain and making its treatment difficult.

In our interview, Jim described to me the day he realized that he did not *have* to overeat. This may seem a strange thing to say, but that is how it felt to Jim. Perhaps others reading this book will recognize the feeling.

Jim realized that, growing up, his parents had always encouraged him to finish all the food on his plate and to avoid food waste. They were not wealthy, and by Jim's account their food was often not appetizing. At some point, he developed an attitude of scarcity toward food; he felt that if he did not seize every opportunity to eat indulgent food and stuff himself to capacity while he was at it, that he might find himself lacking the opportunity to eat good food in the future.

For the 35 years that he ran his construction business, Jim told me, he neglected his physical and mental health. He was not wealthy, and he saw it as his role to put food on the table for his wife and kids. This often meant working long hours and scarfing down whatever food he could get his hands on—sometimes in excessive quantities because he was seeking to fuel himself for the long haul, not paying attention to his body's appetites. Self-care, nutrition, and exercise were not exactly common topics of conversation in his industry.

"You don't get anywhere in the construction business by being a pussycat," Jim tells me. Diet and fitness were often seen by his professional colleagues as concerns for people who were wealthy or "soft," who were concerned about their appearance and who had money to burn. None of these were traits typical of the hard-working, masculine construction worker who had more important things to think about.

Instead, conventional wisdom in Jim's industry was that good bosses and businesspeople work day and night. Constantly pushing himself without pausing to rest or care for his health was, for decades of his life, considered a sign of virtue and a highway to success.

Hearing Jim recount this, I better understood how he got into the state he was in when we met. Eating a whole pizza by himself may have been one of his few reprieves from a life of constant work, or may even have happened unwittingly as he multitasked on spreadsheets while he ate whatever had been placed in front of him.

Finally, after years of pushing himself too hard and eating to cope with trauma, Jim's health had left him physically unable to work. Upon seeing him, I had feared it was too late to turn things around. But despite his excruciating pain and disappointing experiences with medical treatment so far, he was willing to apply his tireless work ethic to a new frontier.

For the first time, Jim's own health had become his priority.

The day Jim realized that he was a successful businessman who could afford to leave food on the plate, he felt as though a huge weight had been lifted from his shoulders. He began to crave less and discovered that eating less made him feel better. Once that positive feedback loop started, Jim had incentive to keep eating healthy portions: when he didn't overeat, he felt better. Perhaps the most important part of Jim's routine, though, has been his dedication to exercise.

Soon Jim was transforming. He began to shed pounds rapidly, and, more importantly, appear more confident. I advised him as best I was able, listening as he enthusiastically related stories of his trainer at the local gym. In time, his previously overwhelming pain became manageable. He started to be able to move around, even doing yard work and taking road trips.

Fast forward nearly 20 years after we met, and Jim has dropped half his body weight. He is happy, a healthy weight, and is now successfully using exercise training and physical therapy to regain his balance and coordination after the onset of age-related neuropathy. Soon, he hopes to buy a new motorcycle. Motorcycles are a passion which he was forced to give up years ago when he became unable to ride one safely.

I am a firm believer that anyone can do what Jim has done. Yet few people *do* accomplish it. Why is that?

Prior to our interview, Jim asked his wife if she could think of any factors that particularly contributed to his success. His wife cited Jim's tenacity and optimism.

"She said that I expect good things to happen," Jim told me reflectively in our interview.

Optimism does indeed contribute to motivation. We are much more likely to pursue *any* goal if we believe we have a shot at really achieving it. If Jim had decided at any time that there was no hope for his improvement, he would have stopped trying.

In Jim's case, tenacity and patience were important too. "This was no overnight transformation," Jim reminds me. Most of his weight loss happened gradually across the course of three years.

"I realized that what I needed was a complete lifestyle change. This was not to be feared, but to be thought of as a gift. With this lifestyle change, I was getting another chance in life. It was fun."

May we all cultivate Jim's attitude of embracing change as an adventure rather than fearing it as an opposition.

Jim notes that his improvement has been "streaky." "Sometimes," he says, "I'll go a while without getting better at my exercises, and then it seems like I'll improve overnight. It's the same with weight loss. I play it day by day. I don't have big goals or deadlines. I just practice every day. I'll get there when and if it's in the cards."

This is another attitude we can all learn from. While results are obviously desirable, preoccupation with our external goals can, paradoxically, often sabotage them. It is our actions and practices, after all, which allow us to achieve results. If we cease practicing because some factor outside of our control causes us not to see the results we want immediately, we can be assured that we will not see them at all. Instead, focusing on our own actions and practices, regardless of short-term results or lack thereof, is the path to success.

"I don't care about looking good," Jim laughs. "In fact, I've probably got 25 or 30 pounds of extra skin under these clothes that the doctors said they can surgically remove. But I don't care. If I lose another 5 or 10 pounds, I'll be happy."

Today, Jim works out two or three times each week with his personal trainer. The pandemic has forced his lessons to become remote, but he has managed to replicate the full range of exercises found in gyms for just a few hundred dollars using something called a "TRX" system—a system of elastic bands and handles which delivers a less technologically advanced version of my home gym's performance for a fraction of the price—a chair which he has nailed to a wooden stand for extra height, and a mirror and webcam to allow him to watch his form.

"Form is so important," Jim tells me in our interview. "If you don't have the proper form in your exercises, you're really robbing yourself of so much benefit. You can feel so many muscles working that you just don't activate if you're not using proper form."

I find this remarkable, coming from the man who was debilitated by crippling pain 20 years ago.

I am not the only caring professional who Jim says has been instrumental to his journey. He described to me his joy at discovering his personal trainer several years ago, who now Zooms in multiple times each week to work with him

"Trainers are important," Jim tells me. "They give you additional self-discipline to carry on day after day. Motivation is more important than knowledge."

Jim has reason to know. "Being in business for myself," he continues, "I had no one else to push me out of bed in the morning. It was all motivating myself. It was tough. It was tiring. It takes a lot of willpower to do that. But having a trainer can actually infuse you with energy. They urge you on. Just asking if you've done your bike ride yet today can make an enormous difference.

"No one doesn't have those 'I don't feel like doing this' days," Jim tells me. "My trainers help me be true to what I'm trying to do anyway."

"He is so gentle," Jim explains. "You see a lot of trainers who become impatient with people at the gym. But he's always checking in to see if you're okay. He built up my routine gradually. Before I knew it, I was doing things I could not have imagined doing weeks ago."

And there was something else that encouraged Jim about his trainer. Jim realized from the start that his trainer was working with some kind of disability. He could not put his finger on the details, and he hasn't asked—but it was clear that his trainer moved a little differently from most people. The man was ridiculously fit, but it seemed clear that he hadn't always had every advantage in the world. This encouraged Jim to believe that he could accomplish similar results, even though he was not the stereotypical young able-bodied athlete.

In addition to a personal cycle, it seems that Jim's success has broken a generational cycle of poor health.

"My father's father died at 58," Jim tells me. "My father outlived his father by a few years." Then, he smiles. "I'm 75 now, and I'm not done or even close."

Though his father didn't enjoy the same long life or good health late in life that Jim has had for the past several years, he did teach Jim a lot.

"One book my father recommended is Napoleon Hill's *Think and Grow Rich*. It might not be obvious how this book is related to health or fitness, but the truth is it's all mental. The book is about mental processes, not financial knowledge. It's about mind over matter. It's applicable to any area of life. Fitness is all mental, too."

Jim has an excellent point there. While the most obvious components of fitness are physical, these physical results are created strictly through mental endurance and determination. The truth is, no one finds exercise to be an easy and simple thing that you just have to *do*. All fitness requires strategy, sensitivity to determine the best solutions for you, and, most importantly, determination.

It certainly was not Jim's physical prowess that has allowed him to get to where he is today; it has been his *mental* prowess. And for that, Jim partially credits Napoleon Hill.

Jim tells me I have also been a source of encouragement in another area of life which he never expected to pursue. This area of life has also been important to my health and wellness journey, which is why I have decided to close this book with it.

"I didn't expect God, exercising, or spiritual life to be in my cards," Jim tells me as our interview wraps up. "If you think I don't know much about working out, you should see how little I know about religion." He laughs.

Jim explains that when he worked in the construction industry, religion and spirituality were often viewed by his peers as topics for the weak. Like self-care and fitness, they were seen as hobbies for people who did not have more important things to do. His colleagues who worked with their hands and their backs and who powered their way through life's challenges the same way one might power through concrete with a jackhammer did not feel that such emotional or intellectual topics were for them.

But as Jim takes stock of his old age, he has become sure that there is a benefit to exploring the spiritual side of life. "If it's coming from the heart," he told me, "it's coming from the right place. My heart is telling me things now. It's very different from how I used to think of myself 20 years ago, when I felt that my role was to provide for my family financially. I didn't have a lot of room to think about this stuff then.

"While all of this was going on, I started thinking about God. Talk about a life-changer. I'm still very uncomfortable speaking openly about religion, but there is absolutely no doubt in my mind that He is responsible for my life changes."

I am not of the opinion that subscribing to any particular religion is necessary to obtain success in health and fitness. But I *do* believe there are mindsets found among the religious and spiritual of the world that can be tremendously beneficial to our health. Several behavioral scientists agree with me.

These ideas are often treated as taboo, both by religious leaders who condemn the "heresy" of interpretations they disagree with, and by secular people who have had one too many bad experiences with self-proclaimed ambassadors of religion and spirituality. Yet science suggests that beliefs and practices which have traditionally been the purview of religion and spirituality can have big impacts of clinical significance on our behavior and our well-being.

We will discuss everything that contributed to Jim's success, from diet and exercise to religion and spirituality, throughout this book.

But first, I want to take a quick look at a controversial question. While some doctors treat weight loss as a cure-all for any medical condition, others argue that a body's size has no bearing on its health or well-being.

Neither of these parties are correct, and both views are potentially dangerous. Let's take a look at the hard evidence as far as how many medical problems are caused by fatphobia, and how many are genuinely caused by obesity.

A Review of the Research

We know that people with chronic pain are more likely to be obese; but does this happen because people with chronic pain struggle to exercise and suffer from a high load of stress hormones which promote stress eating, or does it happen because obesity causes more wear and tear on joints, which can lead to back problems, pinched nerves, and challenges to exercise? Or could it be that both scenarios are sometimes true?

This question affects our decision-making as doctors in a big way. When we see a patient who is both overweight and in pain, which do we tackle first? Do we assume that the extra weight is responsible for the pain? Or do we assume that the pain must be resolved before more exercise and more nutrient-dense dietary choices become feasible?

In recent years, physicians are thankfully more aware of the dangers of fatphobia—a prejudice against fat people which can lead some doctors to incorrectly assume that the patient's weight is the cause of any health problems they may report.

Tragically, it is believed that fatphobia is a contributor to higher rates of morbidity and mortality for fat patients, since some doctors may fail to order potentially lifesaving diagnostic tests for fat patients due to an assumption that a person's body weight must be the cause of their symptoms.

A wide variety of illnesses, including heart attacks and cancer, have been missed in their earliest and most treatable stages as a result of doctors assuming that symptoms like pain, shortness of breath, and overall feelings of illness and discomfort were related to patients' high body mass index. As doctors we must strive to treat all patients equally and avoid unwarranted assumptions about our patients' health.

However, there is also evidence that patients with high BMIs have worse outcomes from a number of health problems, including COVID-19[1] and several other important causes of morbidity and mortality.

It does seem to be true that obesity correlates to higher risks of high blood pressure, diabetes, and cardiovascular disease. What is not always clear is whether the obesity is the *cause* of these conditions, or whether both the obesity and the potentially fatal medical conditions are being independently caused by diet and lifestyle factors. After all, thin people can get dangerously high blood pressure, high cholesterol, and even type 2 diabetes. So it is inadvisable for doctors to assume that fat people have these medical conditions, or that thin people *don't*. Both assumptions can lead to life-threatening diagnostic errors.

In Jim's case, his most life-impacting problem when he first came to see me was chronic pain. Was this pain *caused* by Jim's obesity, or were his pain and the obesity independently caused by a sedentary lifestyle and a diet high in refined carbohydrates?

Let's take a look at the evidence for which comes first: obesity, or chronic pain.

Early evidence may suggest that obesity aggravates chronic pain.[2] One well-known 1992 study showed that women with osteoarthritis experienced less pain after losing weight.[3] Another study in 2004 showed that weight loss in obese women reduced levels of pain and allowed the women in the study to undertake a wider range of daily activities. A 2015 study found that obesity increases chronic pain, and chronic pain *also* tends to increase weight through reduced levels of physical activity and increased stress eating.[4]

According to Stone and Broderick's 2012 paper, there appears to be a linear relationship with chronic pain and body mass index (BMI).[5] Obesity's impact on pain may be explained by the increased levels of inflammatory markers interleukin 6 (IL-6), tumor necrosis factor α (TNF- α) and C-reactive protein (CRP).[6] All of these are chemical messengers which change metabolic function in the body, and all are found in higher levels, on average, in obese patients.

More investigation is needed into why this occurs, and whether this relation is caused directly by a person's BMI or by matters like dietary choices which may be correlated to (but not caused by) both obesity and higher levels of these chemical messengers. Since some of these chemical messengers are known to increase in response to different types of foods, illnesses, and stresses, there is more work about correlation vs. causation to be done.

However, the fact remains that a very strong correlation was found between a person's BMI and their levels of chronic pain. It is reasonable to assume, then, that lifestyle changes which lead to weight loss should also lead to reductions in chronic pain.

Another possible mechanism by which obesity may aggravate or even cause chronic pain is the simple mechanical stress placed on joints when carrying around extra weight. In fact, we know that proteins called "mechanoreceptors," which detect mechanical loads on the cartilage that cushions our bones at the joints, are activated when our joints are asked to carry heavy loads.

This activation of mechanoreceptors in our cartilage leads to the activation of intracellular pathways that result in the production of metalloproteases and interleukin 1 (IL-1). These are enzymes and chemical messengers which degrade the cartilage extracellular matrix and activate inflammatory processes which can lead to sensations of pain and illness.[7]

This all makes intuitive sense. In obese patients, the joints and circulatory system are asked to handle a significantly heavier workload than the body systems of other people.

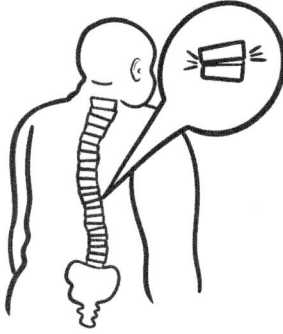

Carrying more weight puts more
pressure on bones and joints.
This can worsen chronic pain.

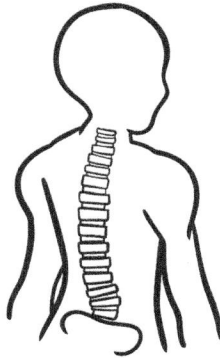

Weight loss can improve chronic
pain by relieving pressure on
joints.

In highly fit people, this may be less of a problem; a person with
strong supporting muscles and a highly trained cardiovascular system
may be prepared to handle this workload without health problems. This
is illustrated in overweight athletes and performers, who achieve feats of
astonishing athleticism while carrying considerably more weight on
their bones, muscles, and joints than most people.

However, a person with poor nutrition and an inactive lifestyle has
not developed their bodies' capabilities to be able to handle this load.
The high workload placed on the obese body in combination with a

sedentary lifestyle that does not maintain muscle strength is likely at some point to result in illness and injury.

However, it is important to be aware that body weight is not the whole story in chronic pain. Many people who are not overweight struggle with chronic pain. While studies suggest that weight loss is usually followed by a decrease in chronic pain, it may not eliminate it altogether. Nor is obesity necessarily the first cause of chronic pain; sometimes it is a consequence of reduced mobility from chronic pain, albeit a consequence that usually makes the chronic pain worse.

We can't neglect the issues that chronic pain presents when it comes to weight loss programs and exercise. Pain is painful. That sounds obvious, but when we are in pain the initial reaction is to remove the pain causing stimulus. If walking causes pain, we stop walking. It is a natural survival mechanism. And indeed, when pain is being caused by tissue damage from mechanical overloading of weight on our joints, sometimes that is a wise course of action.

According to McVinnie (2013), a study investigating activity levels in patients with knee osteoarthritis found that 12.9% of males and 7.7% of females were reaching only the minimum recommended amount of physical activity. Activity levels are unlikely to rise significantly as long as they are hampered by chronic pain.[8]

Additionally, we cannot ignore the impact that nutrition has on both pain and obesity. Pleasure eating is a real issue, especially in those with pain. We know that stress hormones encourage people to eat more fatty and high-carb foods, while discouraging the consumption of nutrient-dense low-calorie foods. Eating is used both as a mechanism to help cope with pain and an analgesic to temporarily reduce pain.

Both pain and obesity can have a multitude of causes. Therefore, reducing pain and body weight should be approached in a multifaceted way; nutritionally, physically, mentally, emotionally. Failure to do so may result in short-term success but long-term failure.

CHAPTER 3

DNA REGULATION

In Chapter 1, we covered the basics of DNA transcription. We explored how the "source code" from which our cells and bodies are built is chemically encoded in DNA strands, which must be copied for new cells and new humans to be created. We discussed the fact that turning DNA into the essential proteins and other building blocks that make up our cells is a multi-step process, with opportunities for our cells to change the way and frequency with which they use different pieces of our source code at multiple steps.

Let us now take a closer look at how our cells can alter our gene expression—and how our lifestyle choices can influence those changes.

HOW YOUR DNA IS STORED

Your DNA is double-protected within your cells. Besides being protected by your cell membrane, it is also covered by the membrane of your cell's nucleus. You can think of this unique compartment as the Fort Knox of your cells. Because this is where the source code that allows the whole cell to survive is stored, it is a very special compartment designed to keep your DNA safe and prevent it from any potential damage or corruption.

A cell's nucleus contains a LOT of DNA. An average human has about *3 billion* base pairs (chemical "letters" in your DNA instructions) and about 30,000 genes (blueprints for specific proteins). Besides genes, your DNA also includes vast "non-coding" regions that do not contain genes but whose chemical properties influence how often, when, and whether the genes near them are expressed.[1]

The differences between different cell types in your body stem from which genes they express. Every cell in your body contains *all* of your DNA, but only the regions needed to make a specific cell type, such as a skin cell or a liver cell, are turned on. Right now, one exciting field of medicine is "reprogramming" cells of one type to become different tissue types, which doctors hope to use someday to help patients restore lost tissues and organs by using other tissues from their own bodies.

This science is still in its infancy. We cannot tell a cell to become a different tissue type by switching genes on and off through lifestyle choices—and that is good news for us. Imagine if you accidentally "told" your liver to become a second stomach instead. Our cells do not listen to us *that* closely because they prefer to keep us alive. However, we can "tell" our cells some things about how we would like them to do their jobs using epigenetic programming. How do we do that, chemically speaking?

Three billion base pairs is a *lot* of DNA, and not all of it is in use at any given time. Unused DNA is wrapped tightly around proteins called "histones" to keep it safe and organized. Imagine a spool of yarn: the histone at the center is the spool, and your DNA is neatly wrapped around it, preventing tangles and knots from forming in the DNA strand. This neat wrapping ensures that your cells can unwind your DNA and use any part of it they might need at any time.

These wrapped up "histones" are organized into larger units called "nucleosomes"—imagine a bunch of spools of yarn all tied together to keep them safe and organized. At the highest level, these spools upon spools of DNA are organized into "chromosomes"—a word you might have heard before. Chromosomes are enormous lumps of histones that are big enough to be seen under a microscope![2]

People with certain disorders have too many or too few chromosomes; this happens because the sperm or egg cell that went into making them experienced a sorting error, receiving the wrong number of copies of a particular chromosome. This can cause changes ranging from unnoticeable (a person may not even notice if they have an unusual number of sex chromosomes, since our cells are made to be able to operate with either one or two copies of the same sex chromosome) to catastrophic (many miscarriages occur because the developing embryo did not have all the genes it needed to build a whole human body).

Take a moment to actively visualize the yarn-spool structure of histones, nucleosomes, and chromosome DNA inside your cells. Read the description above as many times as it takes until you feel comfortable.

See your DNA wrapped up in histones, busy little enzymes transcribing it into RNA to keep your cells alive and healthy.

Now, visualize certain sections of this DNA lighting up. Because you have eaten healthy, or exercised, or gone to therapy, your cells have received chemical messages that the environment is safe. Even the act of taking deep, meditative breaths as you visualize this is helping send those chemical messages. As a result, your cells are turning off genes designed to make you crave unhealthy foods and gain weight. In their place, they are turning on genes to help you relax and have more energy.

Your journey of rewriting your epigenetic programming, which scientists call your "epigenome," has begun.

Turning Genes "On," "Off," "Up," and "Down"

We know of three fundamental chemical mechanisms that determine which of the instructions encoded in our genes are used by our cells and how often they are used. They are:

1. Histone acetylation;
2. Histone deacetylation; and,
3. DNA methylation.

All three of these mechanisms involve the body adding or subtracting chemical groups from histones or DNA. The acetyl groups are the chemical instructions that tell DNA transcription enzymes to transcribe a particular gene differently.

In histone acetylation and deacetylation, proteins in the cells are "told" to add or remove acetyl groups to change the way your DNA spools around the histones that organize it. This acetylation makes the DNA more or less accessible to transcription enzymes, and can determine whether and how often this DNA is used by the cell to make parts.[3]

The proteins that do this may be "told" to acetylate or deacetylate specific histones depending on biochemical conditions within and outside their home cells. Biochemical conditions such as blood sugar levels, specific neurotransmitters, or specific hormones can "tell" our cells that circumstances have changed, and gene expression needs to change also. This is why lifestyle changes such as eating healthy and exercising to lower our blood sugar levels, and meditating and going to therapy to reduce stress hormone levels in the blood, can lead to epigenetic changes throughout our bodies.

When these chemical levels change, our acetylating proteins receive the signal that outside conditions have changed. The cell must now switch survival strategies by altering the expression of genes related to fat storage, nerve activity, and longevity, to name a few. If our stress levels have gone up, changes may be made to increase our responsiveness to fear stimuli (anxiety) and increase the amount of fuel available to cells in our blood (blood sugar). If stress levels go down over time, changes may be made to encourage eating healthy, nutritious food for long-term survival, and to dampen our life-shortening stress responses.

Acetylated

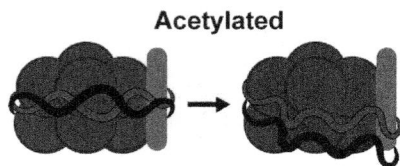

When acetylation occurs, DNA unwinds
and becomes accessible for use by the cell.

Deacetylation

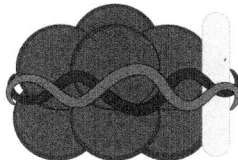

DNA remains tightly wound and can't
be accessed for transcription.

DNA methylation works based on a similar principle. Here, chemical groups called methyl groups can be added to or removed from specific genes, making them more or less accessible to transcription enzymes. Other mechanisms that science is still learning about include histone phosphorylation (adding phosphoryl groups to histones as another set of chemical instructions), chromatin folding (another way to make DNA more or less accessible to transcription), attachment to the nuclear matrix, and regulatory small RNAs and microRNAs.[4] It is possible that each of these regulatory systems is used for different things, allowing our bodies fine control over our gene expression in response to different environmental conditions.

Ultimately, all of these fancy chemical names refer to "tagging" genes with different sets of transcription instructions or opening or blocking certain genes from transcription. Let us focus on the results of each mechanism: each time our cells make one of these changes to our DNA, our gene expression changes. Moreover, by controlling certain conditions within our bodies, we can "tell" these enzymes which genes to turn on and off.

Recall that DNA is tightly wound around structures called histones when it is not being used for transcription. When DNA is tightly wound, it is inaccessible to proteins that aid in DNA replication or transcription. There literally is not room for these proteins to fit between the DNA and the histones. When a histone is acetylated, it allows DNA to uncoil so that proteins can access genetic information. Histone deacetylation means that access to selected genes is closed off; DNA remains tightly wound to histones, and is unable to be transcribed and used to build parts for our cells.

Take a moment to envision this. See the histone without acetylation, keeping DNA so tightly wound that transcription enzymes cannot reach the special instructions contained within the DNA. This DNA will not be transcribed and used to create building blocks of your cells unless something in the cellular environment changes and "tells" the body to use these genes. Let us imagine that the genes in this picture are "good" genes that will make you healthier and happier, but which have been turned off in order to protect you by some personal or ancestral trauma. Let us now visualize them unwinding.

Now picture the histones becoming acetylated. At your commands through meditation, therapy, diet, and exercise, enzymes add acetyl groups to these histones. The histones release their tightly-coiled DNA, opening these good genes up for transcription. The released DNA floats loosely around the histone, while busy transcription enzymes copy the precious information from the DNA into RNA. These RNA copies are whisked away out of the nucleus to direct the construction of new parts your cells were previously incapable of producing. The cell's structure, function, and behavior change, gaining new capabilities.

This is the power of epigenetic change.

Histone deacetylation is often combined with DNA methylation, which silences individual genes. Histone acetylation allows access to genetic information. However, suppose there is a specific gene within the histone that the cell still does not want to use? That gene can be silenced by putting methyl groups on top of its base pairs, preventing transcription enzymes from accessing its data. [5]

Such methyl groups can be added when cells receive chemical signals that a gene is not safe to use under present conditions such as trauma, famine, or illness. The methylation can be removed when the cell receives the proper biochemical signals that this gene is needed or safe to use. If this "safety signal" never comes, the gene may remain methylated and suppressed, even down generations of a family line.

Perhaps there is still a gene on that histone that we just unwound which your body is not ready to use yet. It remains dark and silent, awaiting further changes from diet, exercise, meditation, and therapy to be unlocked. Right now, methyl groups sit on top of these useful amino acids, blocking them. Over time, as we continue to improve our state of health, this desired gene will become unlocked.

You can think of histone modification as a dimmer switch for gene expression, allowing a region of DNA to become more or less accessible by matters of degree. DNA methylation is more of an on/off switch for gene expression, completely silencing a gene when present.[6] Other types of epigenetic modification may have unique characteristics we are still learning about. Still, the principle is the same: in all cases, the cell responds to its environment to "decide" which genes to use and how often to use them.

EPIGENETIC REMODELING

It was once thought that your DNA was your destiny. It was assumed that the body expressed all the genes you received from your ancestors, all the time, in a constant way that could not be changed. It was believed that your inherited genetic make-up was the ceiling of your genetic potential and that there was very little you could do to change your cells' biochemical activity. The idea of "hidden genetic potential"—the idea that we might have genes with abilities we are not using until they are "activated" by making the right choices—only existed in science fiction.

Science fiction turned out to be correct here, just as it has been about so many scientific and medical advancements. For the last 50 years, studies have revealed a growing body of evidence for "epigenetic remodeling"—the principle that lifestyle choices and life events can significantly change the suite of genes an animal's body uses. It has even been found that "epigenetic remodeling" can be passed down through subsequent generations.[7]

At worst, this means that family lines that have suffered trauma for generations can continue to suffer from hypervigilant "fight or flight" responses and the associated biochemical and neurological changes. However, it also means that the actions we take to restructure our epigenetic programming can heal these trauma wounds for ourselves and our children and grandchildren as well.

The field of epigenetics does much to bridge the gap between genotype (genetic source code) and phenotype (the traits that living organisms develop) (Goldberg et al.). For decades it has been known that genes were not the entire story: for example, people with the same harmful, mutated versions of particular genes may or *may not* become sick. Family members with similar genes can show radically different health outcomes. Even identical twins with identical DNA can show different gene *expression*, as read in the RNA that their cells are actually using to build and maintain themselves. How is this possible?

We know that life and family history events change which genes our cells express and how often they express them. Scientists now know that life experiences we can choose for ourselves, and those we have no choice in, can alter gene expression. This means we can get the best advantage for our genes, and for our children's genes if we have not reproduced yet, by choosing to create as many experiences as possible that will turn on the genes we want to see expressed in ourselves.

So how can we use diet, exercise, stress management, and other life choices to change our gene expression?

The first challenge is changing our internal biochemical conditions. We can do this by changing the food we eat and the activities we engage in on a daily basis. This means we must change our behavior. The things we eat, the exercises we do or do not perform, and even our moods and our stressful, enjoyable, challenging, and enriching experiences can all change our biochemical conditions in different ways.

As many of us know, changing our behavior can be harder than it sounds. Fortunately, entire branches of science are available that offer best practices for accomplishing these changes and making them lifelong.

HABITS AND EPIGENETICS

Epigenetic remodeling is a dynamic process through which gene expression can be changed throughout one's lifetime. We can take an active role by using this potent tool to change our genetic destinies instead of being passive observers. The bad news is, a lifestyle of bad habits can also create epigenetic changes that damage both our health and well-being.

Changes to our DNA can be positive or negative depending on how we live our lives. Epigenetics can be influenced by exercise, diet, psychotherapy, drugs, disease, stress, social interactions, and cognition.[8]

We will see in more detail how each of these factors can change our gene expression and how these gene expression changes affect our lives in the chapters to come.

Before we explore specific behavior changes which are good or bad for us, I want to discuss the science of how we change our behaviors. I want to discuss how we can create any long-lasting behavioral change we choose with the smallest possible amount of effort.

CHAPTER 4

BEHAVIORAL NEUROSCIENCE:

HOW TO CHANGE YOUR HABITS

When making health and lifestyle decisions, we often consider every organ system *except* the brain. So many of us have the illusion that everything we do is purely voluntary and that all we have to do—indeed, all we *can* do to change our actions—is simply "make better choices."

However, the reality is considerably more complicated than that. The fact is, there are things we can do to make it harder or easier for ourselves to "make better choices." This fact can hold us back or propel us forward, depending on how well we understand the science of behavioral change and how well we implement it in our lives.

Our brain handles every choice we make. This complex web of neural circuitry, neurotransmitters, and hormones perceives the world through our senses; finds meaning in the sensory perceptions we receive; and decides which information we should heed and which information which we can ignore. Only then does it form recommendations, both conscious and unconscious, for how we should behave.

Our survival is possible because this central nervous system is so complex and processes so much data. Your brain is not only processing an unfathomable amount of sensory data about your surroundings; it is also connecting that data with memories of past experiences, and those experiences are used to help decide your next course of action.

Your actions are also heavily influenced by your biochemistry, such as the presence or absence of stress hormones, the presence or absence of chemical products of fatigue that build up throughout the day, the presence or absence of hormones released when you eat food (different hormones with different effects will be released depending on *what* you eat), and the presence or absence of recent, distant past, or past generational trauma.

If all that sounds pretty complicated, that's because it is. Your body has complex ways of combining all the information it knows about the world, whether through lived memory or epigenetic chemical memory, to decide how you should behave. If your body thinks it is dangerous to waste energy by exercising, or forgo high-energy fuel by skipping that donut, it may well refuse to let you do those things. But if your body thinks that your environment is safe enough that you will live *longer* by engaging in exercise and eating low-calorie, nutrient-rich food, it will happily reward you for these behaviors.

The behavioral science here is about learning what environmental signals to send to our bodies in order to produce the behaviors we want to have. Every tool you add to your "toolbox of well-being" can reinforce all the others. That is why, in this chapter, we will discuss behavior models that you can use to change your behavior, as well as several systems you can use to take control of your choices and change your destiny.

Your body decides about matters like what you should eat and whether to exercise based on factors such as:

Whether your body expects to have to deal with a high-energy crisis. This can be informed by matters like whether you or your parents or grandparents have experienced crises in the past, whether you currently have stress hormones in your body, and whether you have received adequate sleep and nutrition recently or have been deprived, suggesting potentially dangerous circumstances.

The body is more likely to opt for low-sugar, healthy foods and exercise when it thinks you are not in danger of a high-energy crisis. Suppose your body receives danger signals from past or current trauma or stress. In that case, your body may "decide" that the intelligent survival decision is to eat a donut and sit on the couch watching TV to conserve your energy instead.

What are your past emotional experiences with healthy eating and exercising? If you have enjoyed doing these things in the past, your body is more likely to "decide" that they are suitable for you. Suppose you have suffered discomfort, humiliation, or shame around these activities in the past. In that case, your body may decide they are bad for you and "recommend" against engaging in them in the future.

How convenient these choices are for you. Your body is more likely to decide that you should make a healthy choice if doing so costs very little energy. This can be accomplished by planning, such as by taking steps to prepare nourishing foods and exercise options when you are well-rested so that these options will be highly convenient to you later when you are more stressed or tired.

What are some practical ways we can use this knowledge to take more of the actions we want, instead of having our bodies "decide" under the influence of stress hormones that these actions are too costly or dangerous and must be avoided?

As you may have guessed, many of the factors above are affected by our epigenetic programming. Those who have inherited genes programmed to "expect" trauma, for example, may feel that their survival is threatened more by energetically costly actions such as eating healthy or exercising than those of us whose immediate ancestors or personal lives have not known danger or deprivation.

Our genes may produce more stress hormones or produce more stress receptors if we have experienced trauma in the past. This is one reason the work of epigenetic reshaping is so powerful: the actions we take to change our gene expression today can change our body's instincts and responses to stress in the future and make it easier to make the choices we want to make.

As you continue to read this book, you are learning. This means you are creating new neural networks. You are changing your neural processes to promote behaviors that affect your health and well-being. Treatments such as psychotherapy, medication, and exercise also produce changes in brain function at a genetic level, resulting in alleviating symptoms.

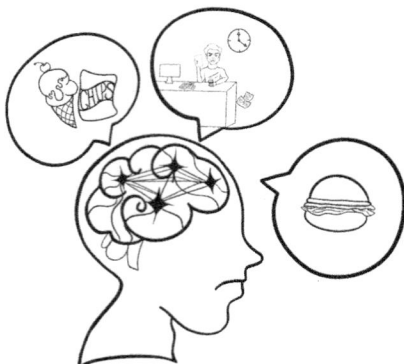

When we are stressed, we
crave unhealthy foods.

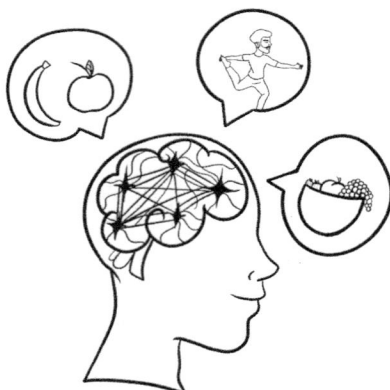

We can form new neural
networks, learning to love
exercise and healthy eating.

TAKING CONTROL OF YOUR CHOICES

Your body's perceived "threat levels" are informed by factors such as
the presence or absence of adequate sleep.[1] Furthermore, nutrition,
the presence or absence of stress, the presence or absence of past
trauma, and the relative convenience of making a choice you want to
make can all affect your likelihood of actually making that desired

choice. To take control of your destiny, you can use approaches such as:

- Ensuring that you get adequate sleep, hydration, and food to tell your body it is safe to fuel healthy choices.
- Planning to make healthy choices convenient in the morning, right after you have woken up and are well-rested. This could take the form of preparing food that will be convenient to eat later, exercising first thing in the morning, or making medical and psychotherapeutic appointments. You are still fresh in the morning, so it's easier to do these things instead of later when you are more fatigued.
- Seeking psychotherapy and other stress management and trauma healing steps to reduce your body's perceived threat levels in the long term and make healthy choices easier each day.

Those steps are helpful, but they are not the *only* practical steps. Because it is not always possible to perform every step on this list, learn and attempt to use *all* the tools in this chapter since each one is likely to fail occasionally for reasons beyond your control.So how else can you make it as easy as possible for your brain to make the choices you want to make?

We have talked so far about how your brain measures threat levels and the wisdom of expending extra energy based on *physical* needs. We have not spoken so far about how your *social and emotional* needs can make it easier—or more difficult—for you to make the choices that will change the expression of your genes.

Recent science has shown that social and emotional needs are just as important to our brains as physical needs. Levels of stress hormones and neurological distress caused by social rejection, fear of social rejection, and other unpleasant social and emotional experiences can be identical to the distress caused by physical injury.[2]

This may be because humans depend on each other to survive. Lacking big teeth or claws, we rely almost entirely on teamwork and mutual support for individual survival. Being threatened with social rejection or social punishment can be just as deadly as being hunted by a hungry lion!

To some of you, this may sound familiar. If you have had negative experiences around matters like healthy food, exercise, and mental health treatment, then the mere *thought* of engaging with these may cause stress and threaten to push you away from these activities in the future. The good news is that you can overwrite these learned responses through a series of gradual, gentle, conscious choices!

For example, you might not enjoy going to the gym because you were teased at a gym or were not taught the proper techniques required to exercise early in life. If this is the case, your confidence may be low, and you may fear social rejection if you visit the gym. This may cause you to behave in such a way that reinforces behavior to avoid the gym. These negative emotional associations may exert pressure on you every time you think about going to the gym, making regular gym exercise feel impossible.

How can you begin to "un-learn" these negative experiences? By giving yourself some positive exercise experiences to replace them! You do this using gradual steps such as:

1. Watch YouTube exercise videos performed by people with a similar body type to your own. Many body-positive fitness teachers can be found on YouTube who show that anyone can exercise and enjoy doing it!
2. In fact, there are books and YouTube channels available from all types of people about their journeys to overwhelming success with weight loss, athletic training, business, family, and more. Fill your media diet with as many of these as possible to tell your brain, without a doubt, that you can do whatever you set out to accomplish.
3. Practice exercises at home to gain confidence.
4. Choose exercises you are confident with for your first gym visits to give yourself an experience of being confident in this place.

This is, of course, only one example of how you can change your thinking and feelings around any activity you wish to engage in more. All-purpose versions of these steps would be:

1. Find examples of people like you doing the thing you want to do. In this age of the internet, where anyone can share their success stories and tips for success, our preconceptions can be shattered if we only look for examples of success.
2. Beginning with easy or convenient activities helps us to deprogram our negative experiences and replace them with positive experiences.
3. To continue creating positive experiences around the desired activity, use tools like social support, favorite songs, and other methods of creating positive experiences for yourself around this activity.

Most of you reading this book have probably tried to change your lifestyle before. You have probably also made excuses for why you cannot or should not perform the action you would *like* to take today or ever again. Maybe it seems too hard. Perhaps you do not have the resources to do it. Maybe today is not the best day. Neither is tomorrow nor the next day.

Excuses may seem like insurmountable barriers. In reality, excuses are valid red flags that show us where we can use the knowledge from this chapter. When excuses arise, our brains bring subconscious objections to our attention. Now that we are conscious of them, these objections can be resolved.

Next let's take a look at some theories you can use to make long-term changes to your behavior.

THE TRANS-THEORETICAL MODEL OF BEHAVIOR CHANGE – THE STAGES OF CHANGE

The Trans-theoretical Model of Behavior Changes developed by Marcus Forsyth states that we go through a series of stages before engaging in a specific behavior. This model has been shown to improve fitness outcomes.[3] We can use this model to understand the best way to support ourselves when going on a life-changing journey, such as improved fitness, making dietary changes, or seeking mental health treatment:

1. Precontemplation
2. Contemplation
3. Preparation
4. Adoption
5. Maintenance.

These stages can serve as a road map to make the best choices to change our behavior. If we can identify what stage we are in, we can take the steps and maintain the action.

Precontemplation about behavior is when the intended behavior is not likely to occur within the next six months. It may benefit you to gather and learn more about the topic at hand during this stage. Start learning about how your life may be affected if you change or decide not to change.

Contemplation begins when the intended behavior is likely to occur within the next six months. It may be beneficial to continue increasing your knowledge about the topic and learning all the benefits of the intended behavior change during this stage.

Preparation involves engaging in the intended behavior in the immediate future—within the next 30 days. During this stage, you convince yourself that this behavior change is aligned with your values and then fully commit to it. This is much easier if you have gathered adequate information to motivate the behavior during the Contemplation and Precontemplation stages.

Action is when the intended behavior is initially engaged and engaged in for less than six months. During this stage, you are taking action, but you may stop if your motivation drops. You want to reduce barriers to continual engagement. It may help to develop strategies to handle setbacks, such as internal or external obstacles. Remind yourself about why you started this journey. Start substituting healthy behaviors for any unhealthy habits that may still be lingering.

Maintenance is when the behavior has been engaged for at least six months. It is no longer a new behavior: it is simply your lifestyle. During this stage, the focus is on preventing relapse. Brief lapses may occur, but you are prepared to handle them on time since you can now draw from a firm grounding of motivation, understanding, and experience.

SOCIAL COGNITIVE THEORY – YOUR ENVIRONMENT AND YOU

Social Cognitive Theory emphasizes the impact you can have on your environment and vice versa. This idea is termed reciprocal determinism. Here, "reciprocal" means that you and your environment change each other, exchanging influences. "Determinism" means that these exchanges determine the outcome for both you and your environment.[4]

This theory simultaneously empowers the individual to recognize their ability to change their environment and cautions them to recognize that their environment will affect their behavior, whether they like it or not. We must make conscious choices about what environments we place ourselves in if we want to have conscious control over our behavior in the long term.

Three factors influence behavior and behavior choices in this model:

1. The environment around you.
2. Your personality and/or personal experiences.
3. Behavioral factors.

In the Social Cognitive Theory model, each of these factors influences one another.

One pillar of this theory is "self-efficacy," which refers to your confidence level in your ability to perform a behavior successfully.[5] The term comes from "self," whose meaning is obvious, and "efficacy," a medical term used to refer to effectiveness and ability to get things done.

A firm belief in your self-efficacy will make you more likely to engage in a behavior. This is because we are more likely to engage in behaviors we believe we can complete successfully than those we doubt will succeed. To create lifestyle change, increase your self-efficacy level—

that is, your belief that you can make changes to your environment and your behavior.

Four sources of information influence self-efficacy.[6] You can obtain all four sources of information to consciously create self-efficacy with careful planning. Since each of these steps positively reinforces the other, each time you take one of these steps, it will make you *more likely* to take additional steps:

1. Mastery experience
2. Vicarious experience
3. Verbal persuasion
4. Physiological or affective states

Mastery experience is the successful first-hand experience in a behavior. When you are beginning an exercise routine, confidence from past experience of having successfully executed past exercises will help you move on to new exercises. This is quite intuitive: if you do something right, you grow more confident that you can do the same in the future, and the likelihood that you'll continue that behavior in the future is increased.

This is a reason to start with simple, easy exercises you know you can do; once you have completed these successfully on a sustained basis, you will have more confidence to add more exercises and continue them over time.

This can be applied strategically in your life by forming and then completing challenging but realistically attainable goals. It may also be helpful to maintain a behavior log to help you track successes and progressions. Every time you meet your goals, you promote sustained behavior, and as we already know, consistent lifestyle changes accumulate over time to show desirable outcomes.

Vicarious experience is obtained by observing someone you perceive as similar to yourself successfully engaging in a behavior. We referenced this in discussing the benefits of YouTube fitness teachers. When you watch a person like yourself succeeding at an action, you can imagine yourself realistically taking the same actions they are taking.

If you see someone who shares the same story as you achieve success, you realize the potential you have to do the same in a way that is impossible without these real-world examples of success.[7] Seek teachers and mentors who once shared your perspective; they know the struggles and techniques required to succeed, given the circumstances.

Verbal persuasion is when others reaffirm your capabilities. It is essential to surround yourself with uplifting friends and family. In-person encouraging communities are the most potent kind. Still, if encouraging people cannot be immediately found in your physical surroundings, supportive online communities can begin building your confidence to seek supportive people in your physical environment.

Words of encouragement offer social support during complex lifestyle changes and increase your confidence in successfully following through with your desired behavior. Never forget the impact you can have on others and their influence on you. One day, you will be the one advising those around you about lifestyle changes. You will provide the vicarious experience and verbal persuasion to the next success story waiting to happen. You can start doing that right now.

Lastly, emotional and affective states influence self-efficacy. We referred to this when we stated that your body is more likely to engage in healthy behaviors when well-rested and not stressed. However, there are also steps you can take to go above and beyond general sleeping and stress management to create positive associations around desired actions in your mind.

When you express positive emotions and experiences, you are more likely to increase your confidence regarding the task at hand. For example, if you are working out in a gym, then smiling, laughing, and enjoying the moment and sensations you experience will create positive associations around this activity in your mind. Therefore, you will want to continue with exercise behavior because your brain knows it makes you feel good.

The same goes for any lifestyle behavior you are trying to implement into your life. If you want to go on a diet, choose a nutritional plan that incorporates healthy food options you enjoy, rather than one that restrains you from your favorite healthy food options. Make a point of taking time to savor how delicious this food is. Practice reframing negative thoughts and fully embracing the process. Your positive thinking and attitude will affect how well you can maintain desirable behavior.

Understanding that change takes perseverance. Each step you take toward achieving your goals is honorable.

THE HEALTH BELIEF MODEL – THE MORE YOU KNOW, THE EASIER IT IS

As you increase your knowledge about your health, you become more invested in making healthier choices. According to the Health Belief Model, learning about health and its impact on your life promotes relevant and meaningful behavior change.[8]

Four components influence your belief about health and its influence on your behavior:

1. Perception of the severity of clinical, medical, and social consequences.
2. Perception of benefits from taking action.
3. Perception of barriers to and costs of taking action influence your likelihood of engaging in a behavior.

First, to help motivate your behavioral changes, you can gather knowledge about potential costs and benefits if you do not change behavior and vice versa.

How significant is this behavior change to your ability to have a successful future? Do you need to be healthy to see your children grow up and get married? What would it feel like to be there for them? What would it feel like to *not* be there for them? How much is it worth making the behavioral changes that make your desired outcome more likely?

These thought-provoking processes help you to successfully take healthy initiative in your life.

Even when you understand the power of your behavioral choices, your perception of barriers and costs of taking action can be a powerful obstacle to adopting the behaviors you want to have.[9]

We referenced these costs and barriers earlier when we suggested that taking steps to prepare for healthy behaviors and make them as convenient as possible when well-rested increases your likelihood of performing these actions.

We can use our daily "hour of power," which will be discussed in the next chapter, to keep the transformative benefits of the behaviors we want, and the horrifying consequences of the behavior we don't want, in the forefront of our minds on a daily basis. We can use strategy to plan for common barriers to action such as family obligations or lack of time, and to combat excuses for not making changes in lives.

That brings us to...

THE THEORY OF PLANNED BEHAVIOR – PLANNING, INTENTION, ACTION

The Theory of Planned Behavior explores the primary influence of intention in determining behavior.[10] Your intention will directly influence your willingness and effort to change or create a behavior. Success will most likely happen once you create a strong intent to go forward with behavior.

Three factors influence intention:

1. Attitude
2. Subjective norms
3. Perceived behavioral control.

Your attitude can be informed by the suggested methods above, including your self-created positive or negative vicarious experiences, mastery experiences, and emotional and affective states. These will work together to form your beliefs and feelings, and attitude toward your healthy behaviors.

"Subjective norms" are social pressures for or against change. If the "norm" in your social circles is unhealthy behavior, you are less likely to be motivated to engage in healthy behavior yourself. Fortunately, you can create your norms by consciously engaging with people who have the standards you desire in your own life. If you cannot do that in person right away, you can seek people who will exert positive social influences on you through online communities.

Last, perceived behavioral control refers to how confident you feel about engaging in the behavior change. If you think this is the same thing as the self-efficacy we discussed above, you are right!

We have now thoroughly discussed multiple ways to improve every factor that leads to behavioral change in your own life. Armed with the knowledge of these theories, you can apply those strategies with great precision.

THE SELF-DETERMINATION THEORY – COMPETENCY, CONNECTION, AND DESIRE

The Self-Determination Theory claims three psychological needs must be met to motivate to start a behavior: competence, relatedness, and autonomy.[11] Competency is interchangeable with self-efficacy. Relatedness refers to a connection with society; find a social support system that works for you. Autonomy is about decision-making based on personal desire rather than externally imposed demands. It is more likely for an individual to maintain a behavior if they perceive it as a choice made through their free will, rather than one imposed on them from the outside.

Once all three criteria are met, an individual will motivate a behavior. Motivation can be described as a dynamic process and a continuum that ranges from lack of motivation to intrinsic motivation, which is when an individual engages in a behavior because they find it enjoyable and exciting.

Every behavior change aims to shift your motivation towards inherent motivation. Once you find the activity rewarding and enjoyable, it is likely you will continue it indefinitely. In contrast, you are likely to discontinue desired behavior if the motivation is extrinsic, such as when you are exercising simply because someone else demands it of you. When changing health behavior, find a meaningful reason for your need to change. This will remind you of why *you* want to make this change, and the benefits you can expect to reap from doing so.

The Hedonic Theory – If it Feels Good...

This theory is based on the premise that the usefulness of behavior or experience is determined by your emotional response to the behavior.[12] If you feel good after exercising, you perceive exercise behavior as a behavior you want to continue. This suggests the need for reframing your experiences and thoughts about a behavior to be positive and rewarding if you wish to continue the behavior in the long-run.

Therefore, try to find enjoyable aspects of a behavior. For example, focus on creating fun and motivating exercise experiences for yourself, or delicious new healthy meals that make you want to eat them again and again.

I know it is unlikely that you will memorize every theory we have discussed in this chapter. That is not my purpose in sharing them. Instead, I hope that you will remember and use the parts which resonated with you when you face obstacles to your goals. I also hope you will consult this chapter as a troubleshooting guide in the future if you find that you are not successful in making the behavioral changes you want to see.

I know that behavior change is possible, because I have done it myself. I hope to support you in doing the same in any way I can.

CHAPTER 5

RETRAIN YOUR BRAIN

We are what we think. All human experience results from sensory stimuli processed through the human brain. Our brains assign meaning, emotion, and priorities to everything around us.

The human brain also learns; it learns what is dangerous and what is helpful; it learns what is pleasurable and what is painful. The problem is these lessons aren't always helpful.

The brain creates memories out of these lessons to keep us out of trouble, and is the reason why the same food or exercise activity might evoke profound positive emotions for some people, and profoundly painful emotions for others.[1] Fortunately, just like our epigenetics, these memories in our brains can be rewritten. All we need to do is make conscious choices to "overwrite" the bad memories we might associate with healthy things with new, *good* memories. We can even overwrite unhealthy memories associated with foods or activities by vividly visualizing the terrible outcomes to which they are linked.

This is a profound insight. The truth is that we have a great deal of control over our thoughts and feelings. We can generate any thought or feeling we wish, at least temporarily. We can create new positive emotional associations with foods and exercises. Although few people are aware that they can do this or even know how to learn to do it.

Healthcare and motivational speaking are two of the biggest industries in the world. Both net billions of dollars each year. This is interesting. The value of healthcare is obvious: it saves lives. However, what is motivational speaking other than someone telling you that it is possible to reach your goals at the end of the day? More importantly, why can you not provide this invaluable service to yourself?

Motivational speakers have sometimes been called "scammers" because the service they provide can, in theory, be provided by their customers themselves without any outside help. Nothing stops us from telling ourselves all the same things that Tony Robbins says. Yet millions of people rave about how hearing Tony's words have changed their lives forever. How is this possible?

Motivational speaking is a multi-billion-dollar industry because human nature is not so simple. Merely knowing a fact or having a goal is not enough: our most important facts and goals must constantly be brought to the forefront of our minds, daily and especially before we make decisions. This principle is so powerful that we are willing to pay motivational speakers billions of dollars to do this for us, even though there is no technical reason why we *cannot* do it for ourselves.

The truth is, we know so *much* that our brains filter out the "less relevant" facts and desires from our minds on an hourly and daily basis. For this reason, we can have full knowledge about a subject and never act according to that knowledge if it is being filtered out and replaced by more immediate—but not necessarily more beneficial—ideas and stimuli. This is why it is so hard to complete the "important but not urgent" items on your to-do list.

So how can we motivate ourselves? How can we ensure that "important but not urgent" changes remain at the forefront of our minds? And how do we keep feeling good while we are making these changes?

ONE HOUR PER DAY

Many motivational speakers and productivity experts have spoken about the "hour of power"—an hour per day, first thing in the morning, in which a person meditates on, visualizes, and takes concrete steps toward accomplishing their most important goals.

The idea is that this hour sets the tone for the whole day: after priming our brains in this way, we spend the rest of our days neurologically primed to consider our most important goals as we make each decision that comes along. We feel great about making the right decisions because we remember that we really can accomplish our goals in this way.

By performing this step *first thing in the morning*, we ensure that it cannot be skipped or procrastinated on. We perform this life-changing step before our other life responsibilities begin to make their daily demands.

This logic is sound. Anyone who has tried to move their "hour of power" to a more "convenient" time can tell you how most of the time, they end up not doing it at all. Indeed, it is by pushing our goals back to a time when they feel "convenient" that we so often fail.

We do not fail because we are incapable of achieving our goals—we are extremely capable of achieving them! Instead, when they feel impossible, it is usually because we have made a series of tiny decisions to deprioritize our goals. These tiny decisions result in the necessary changes not being made. Remember that each of these decisions is completely under our control.

When we fail, it is easier to blame a lack of capability or opportunity rather than acknowledge that our failures are precipitated by a series of small, seemingly inconsequential decisions we make each day.

To ensure your success in this program, I will ask you to do one thing first and foremost: spend between 30 minutes and 1 hour every morning, *first thing in the morning*, reviewing this book and the visualizations and exercises we will create together here.

This can even be done while you are still lying in bed, and it will make a massive difference to the rest of your day. You will make the choices that help you lose weight and gain strength—and you will feel great every time you do because you know you will succeed in reaching your goal!

I said "between 30 and 60 minutes" each morning. Why not the whole hour?

There is some debate about which method is best to keep our most important knowledge and desires at the forefront of our daily decision-making. Some productivity coaches and motivational speakers recommend a single "hour of power" first thing in the morning. Others recommend shorter periods of meditation, visualization, and performing small tasks be spread throughout the day.

These different options may work best for different people. Very busy people or people who do not have privacy throughout the day may do best with a full hour in the morning. In contrast, people who get to make their own schedule or who have privacy in their offices may benefit from 2-3 shorter periods throughout the day. Variations recommended by different productivity experts include:

- The Hour of Power. One eminently satisfying hour, first thing in the morning. During this time, meditation, visualization, and affirmation can be accompanied by simple food preparation, exercises, and taking other practical steps toward our goals.
- One half-hour (or more) of meditation, visualization, and affirmation each morning and at lunch. Some of the world's top performers report that they take an hour or half-hour lunch break, during which they meditate, visualize, and perform small tasks that can help them reach their goals and priorities. This renews their morning focus for the second half of their day.
- One half-hour or more meditation and visualization first thing in the morning and last thing in the evening. Because our brain cements new neural pathways while we sleep at night and can even engage in problem-solving and creativity in our dreams, some motivators recommend meditation, visualization, and affirmation periods first thing in the morning *and last* thing at night.
- The idea is that the brain will better cement our new, chosen thoughts and feelings, work on any problems we may be facing, and deliver any inspiration we may need in our dreams.

There is no experimental research to show which of these approaches is the most effective, so choose the one that sounds most helpful and achievable to you. But remember, virtually all top achievers across industries agree that spending an hour per day, with at least half of that being first thing in the morning, is one of the most important components of their success.

One reason the "hour of power" works so well is that we develop "decision fatigue" as the day progresses. When we first wake up in the morning, we are well-rested and ready to tackle anything (even if it takes a couple of cups of coffee to get there). With each passing hour, we make more and more decisions and perform more and more tasks. Each one tires us out just a little.

As a result, it is harder to make good choices when evening or even lunch rolls around. It is easier to pick a healthy breakfast in the morning than a healthy dinner after a long day at work.[2] After all, why do you throw in that extra bag of cookies when you go grocery shopping after a long day? You may have heard the "healthy eating hack" to do as much of your grocery shopping and food preparation as possible in the morning so that it will be as easy as possible for your future self to eat healthy food.

MEDITATIONS FOR WEIGHT LOSS AND GOOD HEALTH

When it comes to how you can best prime your brain to eat healthily and exercise, I recommend a standard piece of advice for behavior modification: start with the most challenging tasks.

We are going to start our daily "hour of power" with meditation.

What is meditation? Meditation is a period of time where you sit upright (sitting with your back straight helps produce the proper brain activity, in addition to making sure you do not fall asleep!) and clear your mind.

I mean, clear your mind. Stop. All. Thoughts.

This is surprisingly difficult. Sometimes trying *not* to do anything is more challenging than trying *to* do just about anything.

Nevertheless, that is the point. That is why we do this intentionally.

When our mind is clear, our stress levels drop. Our muscles relax. We become more aware of our bodies. We breathe more deeply.

Furthermore, being in touch with our bodies is a crucial ingredient for health.

After we have stopped our thoughts, the other key component of meditation is taking slow, deep, relaxed breaths. Some say you can induce a meditative state simply by taking slow, intentional, relaxed breaths. However, sometimes we can get tense over the question of whether our breathing is slow or relaxed *enough*, which is counterproductive. This is where a Buddhist or Taoist monk would say that the only way we can succeed is by not striving.

Medical journals describe the kind of breathing seen in deep meditation as "diaphragmatic breathing." It turns out that meditating and breathing like this synchronizes brain activity with the activity of the nerves that control the diaphragm, resulting in system-wide drops and stress hormones.

This is so beneficial that it has been found to have clinical benefits for everything from anxiety and eating disorders to COPD, constipation, hypertension, and improving quality of life in cancer patients.[3] The benefits are probably due at least in part to the drop in stress hormone levels, as these hormones can actively inhibit healing and immune responses. Stress hormones *also* tell our brains to crave high-fat, high-sugar, and high-salt foods. The next time you are craving junk food, try meditating for twenty minutes instead of indulging. Both will drop your stress hormone levels, but one will lengthen your life while the other will shorten it.[4]

Meditation pairs nicely with the next thing I am going to recommend. Visualization is most powerful when performed in the relaxed, focused state of mind you obtain through meditation and deep breathing.

VISUALIZATIONS FOR WEIGHT LOSS AND GOOD HEALTH

Visualization is the art of envisioning your desired outcome as though it has already happened. It is one of the most powerful motivators known to humanity.

Some philosophers say that when we visualize something with intensity and detail, we *create* that reality in another plane, which will allow it to manifest in this world if we simply create the necessary conditions for this to happen through our actions. That is not my area of expertise, but I *can* tell you that the more detail you see, feel, hear, smell, and taste the results of your fitness and weight loss efforts, the happier and more motivated you will be to take action to make them a reality.

See yourself with the body of your dreams. See your muscles becoming stronger, your movements becoming lighter. See your body becoming more toned. See yourself looking ten years younger. What does that *feel* like in your muscles and joints? Do you feel energetic and ready to take on the world?

This is all really possible for you. You simply need to take the necessary steps to make it a reality.

We can use some nifty tricks during visualization to change the way we experience future actions. We can visualize ourselves feeling disgusted and displeased at the thought of eating French fries—that is something I have done myself with great success. Alternatively, we can sit and imagine and visualize how crispy and flavorful fresh vegetables taste, until there is nothing we want more than to eat a salad.

This works because the brain creates physical pathways, called synapses, when we visualize a future scene. The more vivid sensory detail we give to this scene, the more synapses our brain creates and the easier it is for us to recall our motivation for our healthy choices.

When we think of ourselves as out of shape, we expect ourselves to behave that way. It becomes much easier to choose to eat healthily and exercise when we visualize the changes we know we can accomplish and behave as though we are *already* living that fitter, lighter life.

After all, we have already inhabited a world where we have made these choices consistently through our visualizations. Now that we have seen what is possible for us, everything we used to believe about our bodies and our behaviors has changed. We create an image of ourselves as that fit, energetic person, and that image is easy to step into each time we are faced with a decision about eating or exercise.

Likewise, when we visualize ourselves experiencing discomfort as the result of junk food, we create pathways between the idea of that food and feelings of disgust and displeasure in our brains. Each time we choose to associate those feelings with that food, we make this link stronger. This can cause the food's power over us to vanish almost instantly when invoking these unpleasant memories.

We can imagine how powerful our muscles will feel as we do our exercises and how invigorating our morning run will be. Instead of associating exercise with a burden or shame, we can imagine how good they feel and how good we look doing them.

Many healthy recipes *are* delicious, so it is not necessary to pretend. If you can't think of many delicious healthy recipes, you may be interested in my book *Dr. T's Drop the Fat Diet* which is available on Amazon. I am not good at eating un-tasty foods, so you can trust me when I say that the recipes in there are full of flavor.

Since many of us have preconceptions that healthy food is less tasty, we can overwrite those preconceptions instantly by imagining how tasty our healthy menu items are and how satisfied we will feel after we eat them.

We can create our reality in all ways, free from any past limiting experiences or beliefs that may tell us that we cannot do this. After all, we can create any thought or experience in our minds even before it becomes reality. And science is telling us more and more that we can create even the ways in which our genes are expressed.

We can. I am living proof.

I invite you to spend 20 minutes or more during your "hour of power" visualizing your most important goals after entering a meditative state. We will finish this period of time with the easiest (because it is the simplest) activity of all: affirmations.

AFFIRMATIONS FOR WEIGHT LOSS AND GOOD HEALTH

An affirmation is a simple statement to remind yourself what is possible. It is a way for you to fight old, outdated beliefs that don't serve you.

All of us pick up some beliefs that fail us in the course of growing up. We pick up a great many beliefs that simply are not true. For example, we might imagine ourselves as not physically fit or as disliking exercise, simply because of one or two early childhood experiences that created the false belief that this was our lifelong state. Affirmations work to counteract any limiting beliefs we have, whether those beliefs are about our career achievement, creative pursuits, or health.

To finish off your "hour of power," you will repeat some of your affirmations while practicing the visualizations and meditative state of mind discussed above. Doing just one is excellent but doing all three simultaneously puts the brain in an incredibly receptive and empowered state.

I suggest using these simple rules for crafting your affirmations:

1. The simpler, the better. Long, complicated sentences may be more challenging for the brain to understand and retain.
2. Do NOT use the word "not" or reference the beliefs and feelings you want to eliminate in any way. "Not" is a tiny word – easy for the brain to miss – and repeating the unwanted ideas in any way can reinforce them.
3. If you are trying to replace a specific feeling or idea, put together words *opposite* the unwanted idea. For example, instead of "I am not out of shape," use "I am an athlete at the peak of health."

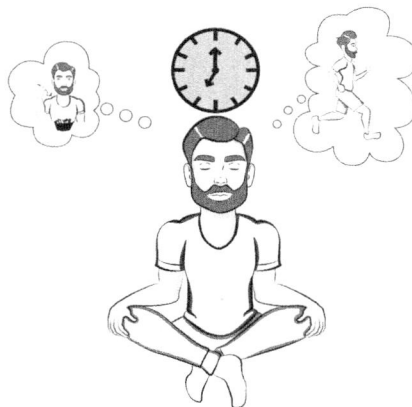

We can use visualization and
affirmations to create the lifestyle
that will get us the results we want.

Here are some example affirmations you can start with:

1. I am an athlete at the peak of health.
2. Exercising feels good!
3. When I exercise, I feel strong and capable.
4. There is nothing more invigorating than a good workout.
5. Fruits and veggies are delicious.
6. I cannot wait to eat some lean protein!

If you feel so inclined, you may wish to keep a journal to track your experience with your "hour of power" – and with these exercises – each day. This will help you be more aware of how your chosen changes affect you.

Does this sound like a whole lot of psychobabble? I don't know what your definition of "psychobabble" is, but I can tell you that this works! In fact, this chapter contains what is likely some of the most universally and directly beneficial material in the entire book.

Still, we live in an era that demands scientific evidence – and rightly so! Anyone can make *claims* about what works, after all. We ought to demand evidence that these claims are true. The more rigorous the standards used to remove bias and obtain accurate evidence, the better.

We will look at a great deal of cutting-edge research in the fields of life extension, biochemistry, caloric expenditure, and more. While we do this, don't forget to revisit Chapter 5 and its exercises as often as possible! Reading about DNA is fascinating, and it might even be motivational. But on its own, information alone will not change your life. Instead, change comes from action; and it is the action that matters more than the information.

I also hope you are revisiting Chapter 5 consistently throughout this reading. Doing your hour of power daily will cause your brain to much more effectively remember all of the information in this book and use it to find solutions to any obstacles you face in obtaining your desired results,

Now that you have your hour of power and your troubleshooting guide, let us proceed to talk about some of the specific physical benefits of specific behavioral changes. We will start with a goal that practically everybody has: that of slowing down the aging process.

CHAPTER 6

AGE AND LONGEVITY: HOW EPIGENETICS

CAN SLOW THE BIOLOGICAL CLOCK

Turning back the clock on aging may not be your purpose for reading this book. You may be singularly focused on weight loss. However, we will cover the epigenetics of aging for one crucial reason: seeing how our gene expression changes with age shows us how epigenetic programming contributes to every critical human discomfort and disease.

We all know at some level what aging is. What we might not fully appreciate is how aging is negatively associated with virtually *all* critical health outcomes. Anything likely to kill you becomes progressively more likely to do so as you get older.

Aging seems to involve a progressive failure of our cells, particularly our body's systems for health and vitality. The biochemical mechanisms of aging *also* affect all the other mind-body outcomes we will work to improve throughout this book. Factors negatively affected by aging (and positively affected by longevity-promoting measures) include:

- Blood sugar
- Blood pressure
- Cholesterol
- Chronic pain
- Weight gain

- Physical energy
- Physical strength
- Mental acuity

Why should these things get worse as we age? Is there a way we can use lifestyle choices to improve outcomes and essentially slow down the aging process, in addition to achieving weight loss, muscle gain, and better health?

Absolutely, yes. Some technologies we will discuss in this chapter are futuristic, but others are available to us today and can be incorporated into our daily routines right now.

The issue of healthy aging—that is, remaining healthy and sharp as the years pass—is more critical now than ever. With birth rates shrinking and life expectancy climbing higher around the globe, the world is looking at a future in which more and more people will be living well into their 90s and beyond, and fewer and fewer young people will be available to care for them.

This may be why the United Nations has declared the 2020s to be the "decade of healthy aging," in which they are encouraging governments, international agencies, and private sector companies to work together to improve the quality of life and the health of older people.[1]

All of this makes it critically important that the people of today embrace age management and healthy aging lifestyle choices, to ensure they will remain strong and healthy for as long as possible. It is clear that the issue of remaining healthy as we age is now of societal, as well as individual importance. Without further ado, let us look at some innovative theories of what *causes* aging and how diet and medicine can improve all the outcomes listed above.

Why Do We Age?

David Sinclair is the co-Director of the Paul F. Glenn Center for the Biology of Aging at Harvard Medical School. His bold claims that the aging process can be slowed entirely, or even reversed, through epigenetic modification have made him world-famous.

As of this writing, Sinclair's claims are considered highly controversial because almost all of his evidence comes from animal studies. Few controlled clinical trials of Sinclair's favorite "longevity-promoting compounds" on healthy humans have been conducted, meaning that at present there is almost no data to tell us whether these compounds work in humans the same way they work in laboratory mice.

This is a tricky area, because medications that have worked well in laboratory mice have had profoundly mixed results in humans. While some medications have produced reasonably similar results in mice and humans, others have produced radically different results. The metabolic differences between mice and humans are not, at this time, well-enough understood to predict whether any given chemical compound will have the same effect on mice as on humans.

For this reason, National Institute on Aging director Felipe Sierra has gone on record saying of Sinclair's proposed treatments, "I don't try any of these things. Why don't I? Because I'm not a mouse."[2]

Still, Sinclair's discoveries in mouse models and yeast cells are compelling. If the mechanisms he has discovered in these organisms do prove true in humans, they could revolutionize our understanding of aging—and of how to slow our biological clocks.

Sinclair's lab has discovered multiple interventions that extend the lifespan of the average laboratory mouse by 40%. If his mice were human, they would be routinely living to 120 in relatively good health.

How does Sinclair do this? His approaches revolve around using diet, supplements, and gene therapy to modify a family of proteins within the cells called "sirtuins." These proteins appear to work by regulating gene function to keep our cells healthy and young. They do this by repairing damage to DNA itself and removing chemical groups such as acetyl groups from the histones that control DNA transcription. Several of Sinclair's most successful interventions for extending lifespan in mice have involved increasing the activity of these sirtuins.

Sinclair believes that aging is caused by damage to DNA—and, specifically, by loss of function in the sirtuins.

According to Sinclair's theory, exposure to DNA-damaging chemicals, radiation, and the simple passage of time causes our cells' DNA to degrade.

Cells suffering from DNA damage experience impaired function and aging.

DNA repair mechanisms help cells function better and appear younger.

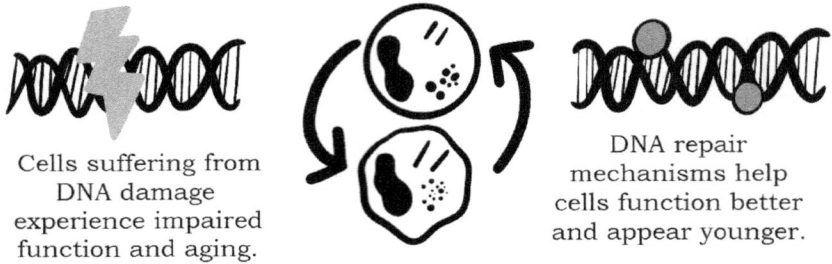

What is groundbreaking about Sinclair's work is that it suggests that this damage is *reversible*. Mice and yeast cells genetically engineered to have extra copies of sirtuin genes, or fed diets that increase sirtuin activity, can repair this DNA damage and live up to 40% longer than their untreated counterparts.

Sinclair's theory is that aging is not inevitable. The information needed for our cells to remain healthy and strong is not *lost* over time. Our bodies just lose their ability to use this information because of a lack of sirtuin activity. If we can turn our sirtuin activity up or re-activate various genes found in healthy young cells, aging can be slowed, halted, or even reversed.[3]

Sinclair believes that groundbreaking longevity-promoting therapies will become available as gene therapy becomes more reliable and affordable. Let us look at the methods available to you right now which might slow the aging process—and how these same principles affect other metabolic processes such as weight loss and chronic pain.

CALORIC RESTRICTION AND LONGEVITY

Calorie-restricted diets are by far the most uncomplicated way scientists have achieved remarkable lifespan extension in laboratory animals.

Around 100 years ago, scientists noticed that laboratory animals that ate about 20% less than was necessary to be "full" seemed to live much longer than animals that ate to complete satiation. In models from yeast to mice to rhesus monkeys, test subjects deprived of 20-30% of their "normal" calorie intake lived up to 40% longer, with the rhesus monkeys in the studies routinely reaching the human equivalent of 120 years of age.

At first, this seemed counterintuitive. Surely not getting enough food must be *bad* for us, right? We need all that fuel for a reason. However, scientists soon realized animals could get all the *nutrients* they need to stay healthy, such as vitamins, minerals, and healthy fats, without eating to the point of becoming satisfied. All that was necessary was a carefully curated nutrient-dense diet and a way to prevent animals from eating that extra 20%

It has been difficult to rigorously test how much caloric restriction increases lifespan in humans because of the difficulty of getting humans to agree to go hungry for decades. It does not help that aging is not considered an acute disease by most health authorities, making it difficult to procure funding or ethics approval for longevity-promoting clinical trials. However, anecdotal evidence suggests that this same principle at work in rhesus monkeys might apply to us as well.

Professor Alexandre Guéniot, a 19th-century doctor who would become the president of the Paris Medical Society at the dawn of the 20th century, had an intuition that eating less might lead to a longer life. He could not put his finger on *why*, biochemically, but it just felt right.

Though other 19th-century physicians often mocked him for his "eccentric" and "unscientific" behavior, he had the last laugh—literally. He was born in 1832; he died in 1935. This is an awe-inspiring achievement, given that almost none of the modern life-extending medical innovations we take for granted today existed at the time of his death.

The effect of caloric restriction on causes and indicators of illness and inflammation such as blood sugar, cholesterol levels, and blood pressure was shown in the study of the experimental subjects who took part in the Biosphere 2 experiment. This group of eight intrepid explorers was sealed inside an airtight artificial ecosystem to prove that humans could survive in self-contained ecosystems in space. Unfortunately—or perhaps, fortunately, in the end—Biosphere 2's closed ecosystem was imperfect, and its residents could not grow sufficient food to maintain a "normal" 2,000-2,500 calorie per day diet.

Despite food shortages and other complications, the crew stuck out the duration of their two-year experiment, eating a calorically restricted diet all the while. After the experiment, they were found to have experienced marked drops in cholesterol, blood sugar, and blood pressure compared to their readings at the start of the experiment. There were known medical explanations for why the body's conservation of energy under calorically restricted conditions would cause these outcomes, but what was interesting was that these findings mirrored the blood work of calorically restricted mice who ended up experiencing lifespan extension because of their sparse diets.

Another line of evidence comes from the island of Okinawa, Japan. Despite being one of Japan's economically most impoverished areas, Okinawa has historically boasted the highest average life expectancy globally. As of surveys done in the 20th century, over 1,000 residents of this small island were over 100 years old. Furthermore, Okinawans did not just live longer; they seemed to age more slowly. As of the 1980s, a full two-thirds of 97-year-old Okinawans were still living independently and did not require help with the tasks of daily life.[4]

Most remarkable of all, we know that this is *not* just a matter of inheriting good genes. Sadly, we know this because Okinawan life expectancies have dropped to match mainstream Japan over the last few decades. Why should this have happened? Well, one reason some scientists put forth is that Okinawans born in the late 20th century are more likely to eat modern mainstream diets while mainly avoiding the island's unique nutrient-dense traditional dishes and philosophies about food.

What is the traditional Okinawan philosophy about food? Well, it is pretty simple: eat until you are only 80% full. Over time, the Okinawans observed that they felt better when they stopped eating while they were still about 20% hungry.

It is hard to know how much this philosophy of restricting calorie intake affects Okinawa's status as one of the world's five "blue zones" where people have historically lived a bafflingly long time for no apparent reason.[5] Nevertheless, the coincidence between the Okinawan lifestyle and scientists' findings from animal experiments with 20% caloric restriction to slow the aging process is remarkable. It is equally impressive that, to the misfortune of the Okinawans, the adoption of modern diets seems to have caused their unusually long life- and health spans to vanish.

If the caloric restriction has been proven to work in mice and yeast, and there is some evidence to believe it may work in humans—why should this be so? What does it have to do with epigenetics?

David Sinclair has some ideas about this. His theory is that caloric restriction shifts the cells' programming and resources away from the reproduction of new organisms and *toward* survival of the current organism. Offspring born into times when their parents are malnourished due to food shortages are unlikely to survive. From an evolutionary perspective, it is better to keep the adults alive until times get better, rather than divert energy toward reproductive functions. Indeed, one side effect of prolonged severe caloric restriction in some women is the cessation of menstruation. The body seems to make a strategic decision to halt reproductive activities and focus solely on survival.

There is reason to believe that this mechanism has an epigenetic basis. Studies of long-lived, calorie-restricted yeast chromosomes found that the DNA of the calorie-deprived cells was wound much more tightly than usual.

This arrangement results from massive epigenetic changes inside the calorie-restricted cells. The epigenetic "off switches" have been flipped wherever possible, winding the DNA up tightly to preserve it and keep it safe. I suspect that a thorough analysis of the calorie-restricted genome would also reveal that specific genes related to longevity and cellular repair have been flipped "on" to maximize chances of living through the famine. The logical net effect of these changes is to considerably slow the rate at which DNA accumulates damage, resulting in a substantially more manageable workload for the youth-preserving sirtuin proteins.

Of course, the logical net result of these epigenetic changes is significantly slowed aging and extended health and lifespan.

Can you, and *should* you, practice Okinawa-style caloric restriction in your own life? The answer is "try it, but *only* if you have a sufficiently nutrient-dense diet." Unfortunately, most mainstream diets are *not* nutrient-dense and require us to ingest more calories to get all the vitamins and minerals necessary to stay healthy.

Fortunately, the eating plan described later in this book *is* low-calorie and nutritionally dense. It can form the first step in a diet that meets your nutritional needs, even as you eat until you are only "80% full."

Caloric restriction using a nutrient-dense diet is the simplest way to potentially address the DNA damage at the root cause of aging and address all the "symptoms" of aging discussed at the start of this chapter.

CHAPTER 7

HOW TO STICK TO A DIFFICULT REGIMEN

So far in this book, you have learned some powerful skills and gained knowledge. You've learned to use the power of visualization to motivate yourself to accomplish your goals. You've learned the science that proves that your goals *are* possible through the epigenetic mechanisms that allow you to change your very gene expression. You've learned some tips to turn motivation into real behavioral changes and learned about the surprising mechanisms that may be available to you to slow your aging process.

But you may also be a bit overwhelmed by this point. All of this information alone is overwhelming; the list of behavioral changes you wish to make, and the list of health and fitness goals you now have, may feel overwhelming as well.

That's why this is a good time to discuss the other most powerful resource available to help you: the resource of social support.

Let's take a moment to use the power of visualization. See yourself adhering to your personal longevity-promoting routine (under the advice of your doctor, of course). Picture yourself enjoying it. Vividly imagine the wonderful feeling of invigorated energy that comes from having a healthy, youthful metabolism. See your mind and your body charging up.

Doesn't that feel great?

Good. Now that your enthusiasm has been renewed, let's try to learn just one more thing today.

WHY SOCIAL SUPPORT IS OUR MOST IMPORTANT SURVIVAL STRATEGY

We are profoundly social creatures. In fact, scientists now know that our social nature is more important to our survival, both as individuals and as a species, than our individual physical and mental capabilities. Teamwork and mutual aid alone have allowed *Homo sapiens* to conquer the planet and survive natural and unnatural changes to their environments. "Going it alone" has never really worked for any human for any meaningful period of time.

You may feel that this is an overstatement. After all, the idea that we should be able to do things by ourselves, without support or assistance, is popular in some subcultures. Some may even claim that this is the more "natural" way to do things, or that this is what our ancestors did in the past. But the archaeological and anthropological records of human history now tell us that this idea is dangerously mistaken.

For decades, scientists struggled to unravel one question: why did *Homo neanderthalenesis,* a species that was similar to modern humans in almost every physical and behavioral aspect, go extinct tens of thousands of years ago while our species was thriving and taking over the globe?

Some proposed that our own ancestors *caused* the Neanderthals to go extinct, either hunting them down or outcompeting them for food sources. But this theory has a big problem: Neanderthals were physically better-suited to win such a war than *Homo sapiens* were in just about every important way.

Neanderthals had bigger brains than us. They were physically stronger, and they were specially adapted to the cold and low-light conditions of Ice Age Eurasia, while our ancestors were fresh out of Africa and had spent a hundred million years adapting their bodies to get rid of heat as fast as possible under the hot African sun.

So how in the world did we win against a stronger, more experienced, quite possibly smarter competitor?

The single biggest difference between Neanderthal and modern human archaeological findings so far is in the size of our trade networks. Our ancestors were aggressively friendly and helpful: both ancient *Homo sapiens* and modern hunter-gatherers today had trade and mutual aid networks that stretched across *thousands* of miles. New inventions and techniques flowed through these networks, rapidly giving our ancestors access to the best ideas from people thousands of miles away.

In times of hardship, modern human hunter-gatherers also use their networks to deliver food and other material assistance across thousands of miles, from people who have plenty to people who do not. It's hard to be sure that early *Homo sapiens* did the same thing since it is almost impossible to distinguish commercial trade from gifts of charity in the fossil record, but we have no reason to believe that ancient humans did not behave the same way as modern hunter-gatherers in this respect.

Neanderthal archaeological sites, on the other hand, show no evidence of such networks. Neanderthal sites do not show evidence of materials from hundreds of miles away, nor did the inventions of Neanderthals in one region seem to spread to other regions. This not only slowed Neanderthals down technologically in a big way: it also suggests that they had no one to turn to for help if their local group ran into trouble.[1]

When it came to human dominance of the globe, this was not a case of the survival of the most physically fit, or even of the brainiest. This was a case of survival of those who were most willing to help each other out. Later in this book, we'll see even more evidence from modern hunter-gatherers suggesting that ancient humans' secret to success is sharing.

This is my long, fancy, scientific way of saying that it's a good idea to be part of a support network in anything you do. This very much includes diet, exercise, and lifestyle changes. Your brain is made to crave a social experience in everything you do. It's made to crave to give and receive advice and encouragement, and to look to others for cues about what you should do. And that is a powerful tool you can leverage.

This may be why even the most successful professionals often benefit from a helping hand. My own age management medical practice includes a coaching component, which has been utilized by top professionals including brain surgeons. One such neurosurgeon gave an interview to a fitness magazine testifying to his experience.

"I wanted to be healthier, but I wanted the process to be as efficient as possible," he recalled. "The program was detailed, streamlined, and enthusiastic. The team gave me direction."

Less than three months after starting my coaching program, this surgeon had reduced his BMI by 10 (meaning he'd lost 10% of his body weight in fat), and he was still feeling excited to do more.

"For me, this has made a huge difference," he reported to the magazine. "I feel more youthful and energetic. It really works!"

One might imagine that a brain surgeon is not someone who is lacking in drive and ambition. However, one might also guess that any man might struggle to keep up the motivation necessary to lose 10% of his body weight safely in three months. The difference between this neurosurgeon and many people who try to reach this goal unsuccessfully was simple: he realized that he needed help. Instead of trying to go it alone on top of his busy career, he found a team of experts to help him.

The point of this story is not to advertise my own coaching services; it is to demonstrate the effectiveness of coaching services in general to achieve our health goals. While many people dismiss coaching services as a useless extravagance—after all, you already *know* what you need to do, so why do you need a coach? The reality is that top performers from professional athletes to Fortune 500 CEOs recognize that coaches help them perform better than they could perform alone.

I know that cost can be a barrier to accessing coaching services for many people. That's why this next section is about how to find or create your own free or low-cost support system.

But do remember: if nothing else is working to help you get the health results you know, hiring a coach may solve more problems than you might expect.

Finding Your Support Network

For optimal support in your weight loss journey, find yourself a team. Find yourself a group of people who will support your goals and who ideally will have similar goals themselves.

This way, you do not have to rely on your own internal motivation. Just as ancient *Homo sapiens* beat the more physically qualified Neanderthals, you can overcome any number of disadvantages by having a strong, supportive team or coach by your side.

This is, in a big way, the driving force behind the success of the billion-dollar motivational speaking industry. People like Tony Robbins succeed by giving you the social support you need from a distance and arranging events where massive social support is offered. At Tony Robbins events, he does not just impart information: he creates a whole tribe of enthusiastic, mutually supportive people who instill in each other the idea that they really can reach their goals.

Now, you don't need to pay a world-famous motivational speaker to coach you to succeed. You *may* benefit from hiring a local nutrition coach or personal trainer to offer you that social support. You may benefit from finding a free or low-cost support group for your weight loss goals in your local area.

Heck, you can do all three if you like.

Motivational speakers and coaches are pretty good at advertising, so I will focus on the third component. How can you find or create a support network to keep you motivated to reach your goals?

For obvious reasons, in-person groups and coaching are usually best. I say "usually" because, as of this writing, doctors including myself are advising against in-person gatherings due to massive surges in the Omicron variant of COVID-19 across the US. This will not last forever. And as a general principle, in-person gatherings are far more powerful: there are many cues and incentives our brains receive at in-person gatherings that we simply cannot receive through a computer screen.

That being said, having only an online community is much, much better than having no community at all to support you in your goals. We will discuss how to find and use both types of communities, with emphasis on local in-person options, which hold much more potential for growth.

Listings for fitness, weight loss, and healthy living groups may be found on your local Meetup, gym, school, and library boards. Facebook can also be a place to find local groups and events, but in your search remember to make finding in-person meetups your primary goal.

When you're looking for groups, remember to look for people who share your own goals, or your own passions. If there is a specific approach you want to take to weight loss, fitness, or age management, look for groups that share those approaches. If there's a certain type of person you prefer to socialize with, look for groups that you would most enjoy.

Once you've got a few groups on your roster, it's a good idea to "interview" more than one group before deciding where to ultimately commit your time. It's hard to predict the true culture and attitude of a group from the outside, so attending meetings of multiple groups and deciding which one you like best is more likely to get you a good fit than just religiously attending the first group you find.

When it's safe to do so, I recommend attending meetings of the three most promising-looking local groups you can find. After each group meeting, ask yourself questions like:

- How did I feel after leaving this meeting? Great? Not so great?
- Did I feel inspired and motivated to continue my journey by speaking to these folks and seeing their results?
- Will I feel more motivated to achieve results if I continue going to this group and making friends with the people there?
- Does this group celebrate each others' results? Or did they seem to be trying to one-up each other? Having friends who celebrate your results is vital to having a healthy weight loss journey.
- Did I see anybody at this group give safety advice? Was it good or bad advice? For safe results, it's important that

support groups approach their topic in a healthy way so that members aren't unwittingly pressured into unsafe routines.

Now, there is also another approach to finding a supportive in-person team. If you have the materials available, you can create one.

Do the people who are already in your life share your passion for healthy living? Is your partner, best friend, or child also interested in fitness? If so, you may gain the greatest benefit from building a support team of your own. When building a good team, remember these principles:

- Celebrate. Getting excited about each others' successes is the best healthy motivation. Tony Robbins knows this principle well; think of his fire walks, where life-changing emotional states are created by crowds of people jumping up and down in joy at each others' success.
- No judgment. The idea here is positive reinforcement, not negative reinforcement. When a culture or group socially punishes people who fail to achieve an ideal, this can lead people to unhealthy or even dangerous means of pursuing this ideal. Alternatively, it can lead people to avoid the pursuit entirely for fear of being judged negatively for imperfect performance.
- Consistency. Meet on a regular schedule that you set, even if you're not feeling in top form. Remember, this is not *only* a place to show off your great results. It is also a place to get support when you are struggling and laugh when you are stressed.
- Laugh a lot. People stick to tasks that they enjoy. Whether you're celebrating a victory or playing an improv game, keep the laughter coming when you're meeting to celebrate your successes and support those who are struggling.

Once you have the power of social support on your side, the likelihood of you achieving big long-term goals goes up dramatically.

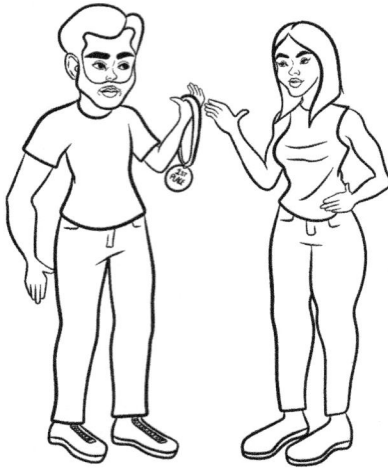

We accomplish more when
we have encouragement
and support from others.

Now that you've learned the second secret to meeting your goals, let's move on to learn more about the science behind cultivating great health.

CHAPTER 8

HORMONES AND YOU

You probably know that declines in certain hormones are associated with some adverse symptoms of aging. Testosterone and estrogen boosters are frequently discussed in nutritional supplementation circles, offering youth-like vitality by restoring youth-like hormone levels.

However, what if I told you that these were not the only hormones which are vital to weight loss, high energy, and longevity? Or that supplements were not the only way to keep youthful hormone levels?

In this chapter, we will look at a brief run-down of the six hormones in our bodies that are *most* important to aging-related factors such as diet, stress, cellular repair, and sleep. We will look at how diet, exercise, and stress affect each of these hormones to produce a truly comprehensive picture of *why* these lifestyle choices might make us look and feel better and why it might make sense for our bodies to use these hormones to "tell" our cells whether to act older or younger.

Longevity experts do not always agree about the best way to slow aging. Nevertheless, they *do* usually come to conclusions that mirror age-old wisdom about healthy habits. David Sinclair and Nobel prize winner Elizabeth Blackburn disagree on the importance of telomerase in aging, for example. However, both agree that healthy sleep, vegetable consumption, and stress management are essential to beating the biological clock.

Blackburn's 2009 Nobel prize was awarded for discovering how telomerase—an enzyme that repairs structures at the end of chromosomes called "telomeres"—can protect our DNA from age-related damage. Blackburn and her lab partners, Carol W. Greider and Jack W. Szostak, discovered that these regions of our DNA are composed of non-coding, repeating DNA sequences—essentially "extra" DNA—which act, in one famous metaphor, "like shoelace caps," protecting the vital DNA within our chromosomes from unraveling.[1]

In Blackburn's research, cells with longer telomeres "acted" younger. Those with shorter telomeres showed more signs of aging and age-related damage. Telomere length shortened in all cells over time. This has led Blackburn and others to conclude that telomere shortening is a primary *cause* of aging. Food and activities that stimulate the telomere-repairing enzyme telomerase can slow down or reverse the aging process. Telomerase adds more DNA to the telomere "shoelace caps," making them longer and increasing our chromosomes' protection from some forms of age-related damage. This idea left scientists of the late 20th century scrambling to find supplements and medications that would "turn on" telomerase, hopefully reducing or reversing age-related DNA damage and reversing the aging process itself.

In her 2017 book *The Telomere Effect*, Blackburn and her coauthor, the psychologist Elissa Epel, make an even more shocking and far-reaching claim. Not only are telomeres a vital controller of the aging process, but physical and psychological stress *shortens telomeres*. According to Blackburn and Epel's studies of people with stressful life conditions, such as people living in poverty and mothers caring for seriously ill children, people who live in stressful circumstances have shorter telomeres, which may be one reason people who suffer stress and trauma rarely live as long as those with easier lives.

Blackburn and Epel subsequently put forth a startling hypothesis: if people can take measures to reduce stress in their lives, appreciate the surrounding beauty, and get plenty of sleep, they can slow down damage to their telomeres and slow down the aging process.[2]

David Sinclair is not so sure that Blackburn is right about the primary mechanism of aging. He and other aging scientists, such as Judith Campisi of the Buck Research Institute for Aging, believe that telomere shortening is a *symptom* rather than a *cause* of aging. Since Blackburn's primary study area is telomeres, it is natural for her to focus on these. What she is seeing might be an *effect* rather than a root *cause* of aging.

Sinclair notes shortened telomeres were one of many symptoms of aging he saw in animal cells because of insufficient activity of the DNA-repairing sirtuin enzymes. He believes that low sirtuin activity is the actual root cause of aging and notes that measures shown to increase telomere length in the lab are *also* shown to increase sirtuin activity.

Judith Campisi believes telomeres are probably not the root cause of aging but a symptom. If reversing aging were as simple as lengthening the telomeres, Campisi believes, scientists would have learned how to reverse aging decades ago.[3]

However, these scientists agree on a few essential truths:

1. Particular lifestyle and diet choices can slow down overall aging and all of its signs and symptoms.
2. People and animals who adopt these choices tend to live longer, healthier, happier lives.
3. Certain fruits and vegetables contain chemicals that help slow down aging. Getting enough sleep and practicing stress management also seem to slow the aging process.

It would be easy to simply list the lifestyle interventions that are thought to slow the aging process. We have already listed some of them in early chapters. However, since this book is about understanding the science behind weight loss, aging, and other health factors, I want to use this chapter to discuss the role of several vital hormones in the aging process.

Leaping from telomeres to hormones might seem like quite the conceptual leap. After all, what do our hormones have to do with the length of the telomere "shoelace caps" that protect our DNA from age-related damage? As Sinclair and Campisi point out, the root causes of telomere shortening and aging are not always clear. All the causes of aging discussed by Sinclair, Blackburn, and others are *also* correlated to hormone activity.

How can this be so? Well, hormones are nothing more or less than the body's chemical messengers. Hormones travel through the bloodstream, "telling" cells across the body how to function. Scientists are only just beginning to understand their profound impact on every aspect of our health and metabolism. At least half a dozen hormone messengers are at work in our bodies telling our cells how to process the food we eat, what chemicals to make, and when and whether to produce new, healthy tissues.

Our hormones are part of the chemical messaging system that "tells" our bodies how our longevity-promoting and DNA-repairing sirtuin enzymes should respond to forces such as diet, psychological and physiological stress, and exercise.

Sounds pretty important, right?

Despite the importance of hormones to longevity and overall health, I want to note here that I do *not* advocate using artificial hormone supplements or hormone replacement therapy for otherwise healthy people. Why is that?

There are at least six crucial hormones that have significant effects on our body's healing, growth, and aging processes. Our body knows how to modulate the levels of all six in a way that is appropriate for our overall health state and lifestyle. Simply pumping extra hormones may be like trying to repair a marvelously delicate and complex Swiss pocket watch with a sledgehammer. More power is not always better, especially for our bodies, which accomplish remarkable outcomes like good health and long life by being finely tuned chemical machines.

You would not put a Formula One turbocharged race car engine into a classic car. While technically an excellent way to gain speed, this extra speed without other upgrades to the car's skeleton or tires would rip the vehicle apart from the inside, eventually resulting in catastrophic system failure and the destruction of the beautiful and valuable vehicle. This is, in fact, not an inappropriate metaphor for what happens to overenthusiastic users of hormone supplements.

To date, as far as I know, no hormone supplement perfectly balances and regulates these powerful forces in a way that results in increased health and longevity over the long term. While these extra hormones may technically achieve the desired effects, they are not balanced or monitored by the body's genetic mechanics and can quickly cause more problems than they solve.

Therefore, instead of artificially pumping hormones into our bodies, it is a better idea to tell our internal cellular mechanics—our "pit crew," if you will, composed of enzymes like sirtuins and telomerase— what results we wish to achieve in this year's racing season. They know how to achieve these results better than we over-enthusiastic car fans who know only that we enjoy both our '63 Ferrari 250 GTO body and the speed and strength of a Formula One race car engine. This is one place where amateur tinkering is not likely to end well.

Next, I will explain how our everyday choices about eating, sleeping, and exercise will *naturally* "tell" your body to make hormone production choices that keep you younger longer, besides many other health benefits.

Insulin: Or Why Sugar is So Bad for You

Insulin has been described by Jason Fung, M.D., author of "The Obesity Code," as the hormone that makes us fat.[4] This is quite true. Although it is essential for our survival as the enzyme that allows our cells to open the cap of their gas tanks and refuel, too much of it can cause our cells to *overfill*. Our cells' fuel tanks are elastic, unlike a car's gas tank, so letting in too much fuel results in weight gain and many unpleasant complications.

This is not precisely how insulin works at a chemical level, but it is an apt enough metaphor to explain why patients treated with insulin often develop progressive weight gain. It turns out to explain why people who eat a lot of sugar and refined carbohydrates *also* gain weight: eating sugar and refined carbs *causes* insulin to be released into the blood. The body's logic seems to be this:

1. Fuel—blood glucose—is present in large, accessible quantities.
2. We must store as much fuel as we can in case fuel is scarce tomorrow. Release the insulin to open the gas tanks!
3. When the fuel is not immediately used, it is converted into fat for long-term storage.

Over time, overexposure to blood sugar causes the body to realize that it may not *need* to store fuel quite so aggressively since the blood always seems to be saturated with sugary energy. So perhaps the cells do not need to respond when moderate amounts of insulin are released; maybe they can wait until insulin and blood sugar levels are high to open their gas tanks to refuel.

This learned response, called "insulin resistance," leads to even more devastating consequences such as type II diabetes. Carried to the extreme, insulin resistance can cause lethally high blood sugars. Cells' refusal to take up sugar from the blood, combined with a high-carb diet, can cause blood sugar levels to rise so high as to cause blindness, tissue death, kidney failure, coma, and death.

Insulin resistance can develop even in people who may not initially gain lots of weight.[5] Therefore, it is essential to have your blood sugar and A1C levels checked regularly by your doctor, as these will show you if your cells are still taking up blood sugar healthily or letting sugar build up in the blood to dangerously high levels.

One of the biggest revelations of recent metabolic science has been discovering the critical role insulin plays in most people's weight loss and weight gain. As it turns out, it is not only how *much* you eat that determines your weight loss or weight gain and your blood sugar levels. Refined sugar and other refined carbs cause blood sugar and insulin levels to skyrocket much higher than other foods that slowly release sugar into the blood.

The *worst* foods for promoting weight gain and insulin resistance, which can prompt massive blood sugar and insulin spikes when eaten, include:

- Any kind of refined sugar.
- Other highly refined carbohydrates including white flour, white bread, most pasta, and white rice.
- The extreme effect of these foods on blood sugar—and the extreme effect of blood sugar on weight loss, insulin resistance, and general organ functioning—is the reason none of these items appear in my weight loss and longevity diet plan *at all*.

Much *better* foods that release glucose slowly over time, keeping blood sugar and insulin levels low, include:

- Vegetables and fruits. As a bonus, many of these are also packed with other longevity-promoting chemical precursors.
- Plant-based fats and proteins, such as nuts, beans, and other legumes.
- Complex carbohydrates break down slowly in the body, releasing low sugar levels over time, such as root vegetables, whole grain and brown flour, bread, pasta, and rice.
- Animal proteins and fats (though some longevity experts like David Sinclair recommend these to be eaten in small amounts).

These healthy foods don't raise insulin levels sharply like refined carbohydrates do, and fewer insulin spikes can mean weight loss.

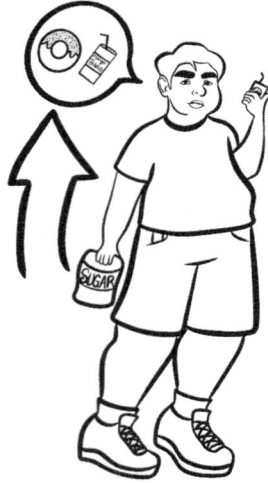

When we consume sugar
and refined carbohydrates,
our insulin levels go up.
This leads to fat storage.

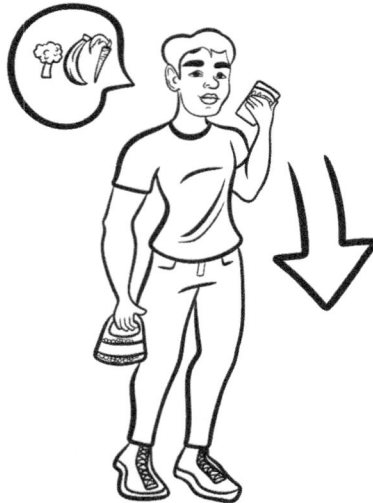

When we eat complex
carbohydrates instead, our
insulin levels do not spike
and our bodies do not store
fat.

It is worth noting that David Sinclair's most powerful life-extending suggestions, such as caloric restriction and intermittent fasting, are *also* recommended by Jason Fung for weight loss, blood sugar management, and overall metabolic health. It seems that keeping our blood sugar and insulin levels low through our choices of what, when, and how much we eat has myriad metabolic benefits for longevity, cosmetics, and overall health.

Also interestingly, metformin—the leading medication prescribed to lower and stabilize blood sugar in non-insulin-dependent diabetics—is also one of David Sinclair's favorite longevity-promoting drugs. This suggests there may be a deep connection between the mechanism by which metformin manages blood sugar and how our cells age.

Nevertheless, as with hormone supplementation, do not just take the medication and assume you do not need to do anything else. There are countless reasons to avoid refined carbohydrates over and above the risks of acutely elevated blood sugar, such as activating DNA-repairing longevity-promoting sirtuins.

CORTISOL

Cortisol is popularly known as "the stress hormone." While many scientists point out that this is an oversimplification of its essential role, cortisol levels are raised by emotional and psychological stress—chronically high cortisol levels make almost every major threat to our health and youthfulness much, much worse.[6]

Cortisol is released by the body when it thinks we are in acute danger. It is released in the wild when we realize there may not be enough food to get through the winter or a lion is stalking us.

In these circumstances, the effects of cortisol make sense. Cortisol's effects within the body include:

- Increasing blood sugar
- Decreasing our body's immune system and healing responses
- Increasing blood pressure

- Decreasing digestion of food
- Keeping us awake

If you are about to be running from a lion or facing famine conditions, this response is a good thing! Increased blood pressure and blood sugar supercharge your cells' fuel tanks, delivering more food and oxygen to combine into bursts of speed and strength. Diverting energy from immune function, wound healing, and digestion saves energy to survive a famine or a fight-or-flight situation. Keeping us awake and alert helps us to avoid danger.

You may notice a significant overlap between these effects of cortisol and the standard health and longevity problems experienced by modern people. That is because many of our current health problems can be traced directly to stressful lifestyles making our cortisol levels too high (that, plus sugary refined food diets).

Unfortunately, in the modern world, cortisol is released in response to stimuli such as emails or reprimands from our bosses, relationship stress, career worries, financial worries, F.O.M.O., social-media-related stress...you get the idea. In the modern world, cortisol triggers are everywhere. Furthermore, none of them require running from a lion to survive. None of them benefit from having higher blood sugar or less sleep. Quite the opposite is true.

Cortisol's role in boosting blood sugar, cutting back on bodily repair responses, and interfering with sleep may be among the reasons Dr. Blackburn found that people with severe chronic stress had shorter telomeres and did not live as long. Some of these effects can be offset with a healthy diet, making it harder for blood sugar to rise to dangerous levels. One can see how cortisol could make the effects of an unhealthy diet even worse by telling the body to boost its blood sugar levels as though you were in a starvation situation.

Cortisol and cortisol promoters *are* sometimes used therapeutically in situations where their effects are acutely helpful. For example, people with overenthusiastic immune and inflammatory responses may prescribe cortisol-promoting medications to suppress these overenthusiastic responses.

For most of us, though, lower cortisol levels mean better health. My prescription to lower cortisol includes components like:

1. Limiting work- and relationship-related stress. While you may feel it is impossible to eliminate these from your life, consider longevity, weight loss, and improved health to be different reasons to follow your therapist's advice to be educated and disciplined about making boundaries and enforcing them.

2. Measures such as cutting back on time spent on the internet and with stressful people can have a tangible impact on your health, in part through the powerful mechanism of cortisol release. Limit the options to ruin your day with stressful work-related emails or social media messages as much as possible.

3. Pursue warm, supportive relationships, communities, and social interactions. The most extensive study of longevity to date found that *the single most powerful predictor* of long lifespan was a person's frequency of warm, affectionate, social interactions. This did not even mean people who were famous or had prominent, happy families: those who lived longest even engaged in warm, genuine connections with their supermarket clerks and bank tellers.

4. Get enough sleep. While elevated cortisol levels can *cause* a lack of sleep, chronic lack of sleep can also impair brain function, making everyday life feel more stressful and boosting levels of neurotransmitters associated with stress. In this chicken-and-egg problem, simply allowing yourself to catch up on sleep is an easy first step toward lower stress levels and better health—even for the lazy among us![7]

ESTROGEN

Estrogen helps keep us young. Where estrogen is found, at least some cells in the body heal and repair themselves faster while making more youthful proteins such as collagen that keep our skin muscles more solid and resilient, it keeps our bones strong and helps to keep our blood vessels healthy. Estrogen even plays a role in the speed at which wounds heal.[8]

Both men and women's bodies contain estrogens in their younger years, though estrogen's role in triggering secondary sex characteristics means that women have more of it than men in their youth.

In the past, estrogen supplements have been given to women to stave off signs of aging. This proved to be a mistake for most patients, as estrogen in high levels proved to increase the risk of serious blood clots and stimulate the growth of certain types of cancer cells, as well as causing other imbalances in the body.[9]

Adding natural estrogen to an aging body turned out to be a bad idea. However, we can still eat fruits and vegetables that naturally help our body make estrogen while simultaneously staving off age-related DNA damage using the techniques we discuss here.

Low-carb diets and low-stress lifestyles can slow down damage to our DNA. Now, what foods can help increase estrogen levels naturally?

Phytoestrogen is an estrogen-like hormone found in plants. Inside the human body, it can have a similar effect to estrogen and serve as raw material for the production of human estrogen.[10] Because women have naturally higher estrogen levels than men, it is sometimes recommended that men avoid consuming too *much* of these plants. However, the medical research is divided over whether consuming these plants causes health problems or any visible "feminization" in men.[11]

Plants that are high in phytoestrogen include:

1. Soybean products include soybeans, soy milk, miso, tempeh, and tofu.
2. Seeds such as flaxseeds, sunflower seeds, sesame seeds, almonds, and walnuts.
3. Fruits such as apples, pomegranates, strawberries, cranberries, and grapes.
4. Vegetables such as carrots, yams, lentils, mung beans, alfalfa, and other sprouts.

5. Plant-based drinks, including coffee, bourbon, beer, red wine, and olive oil. Red wine also contains resveratrol, a chemical touted by David Sinclair as a critical longevity-promoting compound.
6. Grains include oats, barley, and wheat germ.
7. Herbs, including red clover, licorice root, and hops. People who consume large amounts of these herbs should research their cautions, warnings, and drug interactions. Many herbs contain bioactive chemicals that can cause complications in large doses. Licorice root, for example, contains an enzyme that can affect heart rhythm in dangerous ways in large doses or if taken with certain medications.

Another important class of hormone-related plant compounds is indoles, which are believed to have longevity-promoting properties and specifically prevent the spread of hormone-related cancers in both men and women.

People eating a diet high in phytoestrogen may wish to load up on indoles as well. Foods high in indoles are also among those foods recommended by David Sinclair as part of his longevity-promoting regimen and considered among the healthiest foods in the world.

Foods high in cancer-fighting indoles include:

1. Brussels sprouts
2. Broccoli
3. Bok choy
4. Cabbage
5. Turnips

TESTOSTERONE

Testosterone is another hormone that promotes youthful body function, and its levels gradually fall with age. Just as women have more estrogen than men, men have more testosterone than women. However, just as with estrogen, *some* testosterone is found in both sexes and is necessary for healthy and youthful functioning. For this reason, men may especially wish to load up on testosterone-producing activities—but women need not shy away from these, either.

Just as with estrogen, artificial supplementation with testosterone has been tried to stave off aging in men. However, as with estrogen, these therapies have been found to have potentially dangerous medical complications in otherwise healthy people.[12] Like cortisol and estrogen, doctors may sometimes prescribe testosterone supplementation to treat specific problems. However, unregulated, over-the-counter testosterone supplements should be avoided, and otherwise, healthy men with normal testosterone levels are unlikely to benefit from prescription testosterone therapy.

In healthy amounts, testosterone promotes muscle growth, sex drive, and increases energy levels. Too much testosterone can cause aggressiveness, irritability, acne and can cause excess hair growth in women. Testosterone production naturally falls in both men and women beginning in middle age.

Those seeking to increase testosterone naturally as part of a longevity-promoting lifestyle regimen may be surprised to hear the top ways to accomplish that goal. These include:

1. Exercise and lifting weights. In both sexes, exercise, especially weight-bearing exercise, increases testosterone levels in older people. This may be related to testosterone's role as a promoter of muscle growth. When we "tell" our bodies that we need to build more muscle, they may release testosterone. Muscle mass also has benefits for fat loss and blood sugar.

2. Eat healthy fats. Testosterone is made from fatty precursor chemicals, so eating too *little* fat can impair the body's ability to produce testosterone. That is one more reason fat-free diets are not the healthiest; instead, diets that include a nourishing blend of natural plant fats, complex carbs, and plant protein seem to help people live the longest.

3. Reduce stress. It turns out that stress can decrease testosterone levels through several mechanisms related to the effects of stress on diet and other aspects of metabolism.

For that reason, stress reduction is one of the top ways to increase testosterone naturally![13]

MELATONIN

We have mentioned the vital role of sleep several times. To quote Shakespeare, sleep truly does "knit up the raveled sleeve of care." In fact, during sleep, the body undergoes biochemical processes that strengthen our immune systems, repair physical damage, and regulate levels of health-sustaining hormones and mood-influencing neurotransmitters.

Sleep is also *caused* by one specific hormone called melatonin. Our brain releases melatonin in response to many influences, including levels of other hormones and levels of light throughout the day. As with estrogen and testosterone, melatonin production decreases with age if lifestyle steps are not taken to keep melatonin production going strong.

Our body's melatonin monitors use light levels to ensure that we sleep at night and are awake during the day. These chemical receptors are susceptible to blue light, most abundant in the morning and afternoon when the sun is high in the sky. Many apps and other products offer to reduce the levels of blue light produced by our computer and phone screens, which may otherwise confuse our bodies into thinking it is morning or midday even as night approaches!

Besides ensuring we get healthy sleep, melatonin is a powerful antioxidant that may directly prevent age-related damage within our cells. Melatonin's antioxidant activity, combined with correlations between melatonin levels and immune and healing functions (which may or may not be caused by the role of melatonin in getting healthy sleep), have caused melatonin to become a topic of discussion age management and life extension circles.[14] Several recently published papers suggest that melatonin supplementation should be studied to slow down the aging process and potentially extend life.[15]

Melatonin's effect on immune function is so strong that melatonin supplementation was discussed as a preventative measure early in the COVID-19 pandemic after one doctor noticed that patients taking melatonin supplements seemed significantly less likely to die of the disease. Whether that was due entirely to melatonin's sleep benefits and sleep's benefits to the immune system or another biochemical mechanism is unknown.

Melatonin supplements are available over the counter in most pharmacies, and these are believed to be less dangerous than over-the-counter replacements for estrogen and testosterone. However, one caution is that taking melatonin supplements may impair the brain's ability to produce melatonin without supplementation since artificially raising melatonin levels sends the message that the brain does not need to make more melatonin on its own. For that reason, improving the brain's melatonin production through lifestyle choices may be preferable to buying a supplement.

Natural ways to improve melatonin production include:

1. Avoid light exposure, especially to blue light, at night. Avoiding screens altogether for at least two hours before bed is ideal for stress management and sleep quality. If that cannot be done, use blue light filter apps.
2. Drop your core temperature. Getting out of a warm bath shortly before bed or sleeping in a cool room can help signal to your body that the temperature is dropping, signaling the transition from day to night. Sleeping in a cool room has improved overall sleep quality, and longevity experts believe that warm baths and cold showers may trigger life-extending stress reactions throughout the body.
3. Melatonin and the raw materials to help your body make it can be found in foods including milk, grapes, cherries, strawberries, seeds, legumes, and nuts. Pistachios are exceptionally high in melatonin.
4. You may notice a significant overlap between high-melatonin foods and foods that make our "healthiest foods list" for other reasons, such as phytoestrogen or longevity-promoting chemicals. These foods factor heavily in the recipes in my *Dr. T's Drop the Fat Diet* book.

GROWTH HORMONE

Another hormone you may hear frequently mentioned in longevity-promoting medicine and lifestyle discussions is growth hormone (G.H., or HGH for "human growth hormone"). I want to take a moment to discuss this hormone here, as there is a great deal of misinformation being spread by unscrupulous supplement companies.

In young people, growth hormone promotes the development of bone and muscle mass. It's another hormone that usually decreases as we get older.[16] As with other hormones, some people suggest we take artificial growth hormones to reverse aging and gain strength and vitality.

There is some modest evidence that taking Human Growth Hormone may slightly increase muscle strength and muscle mass in men. However, these studies do not make it clear how much of the increased "muscle mass" is muscle fiber vs. excess water weight which may not be healthful, and they do show that muscle fibers under the influence of HGH do not behave more "youthfully" in terms of healing and regeneration.

Artificial supplementation with HGH may be linked to excessive fluid retention, high cholesterol and increased heart disease risk, certain cancerous tumors, blood sugar problems, and in some cases the growth of breast tissue in men.[17]

As such, the medical community has debated the risks vs. benefits of prescribing HGH for older men who suffer safety risks as a result of sarcopenia and muscle frailty. So far, no consensus on whether such a treatment would have net benefit has been reached. And one thing is certain: this hormone is not a "fountain of youth" as some advertisements would suggest. In fact, it appears to have very little to do with youth at all.[18]

What do scientists recommend that people who want to stay young do instead of taking human growth hormone? The prescription is simple, and thanks to our discussion in this book, you now have a thorough biochemical idea of *why* these prescriptions work:

- Exercise regularly, preferably with moderate-intensity exercise, for at least 30 minutes, at least three days per week.
- Eat a healthy diet rich in hormone-boosting fruits and vegetables, as well as lean proteins and plant-based fats.
- Get plenty of sleep, preferably during the same time window each night. Sleeping reliably at night will boost melatonin production, immune functions, and your body's natural healing processes.

How can we eat in a way that helps us naturally boost our hormone levels and metabolic activity to our younger selves? Let's find out!

CHAPTER 9

HOW TO EAT HEALTHY EVEN WHEN YOU'RE STRESSED

We have now seen exactly how important our diet is to our bodies. By virtue of our food, we can affect our gene expression, the rate at which our bodies age, and our overall hormone levels. By choosing what we put into our bodies, we can precisely determine what we get out of them.

The problem is that dieting is hard. Like, really hard.

Maybe you have already been breezing through your chosen diet as you read this book. If so, more power to you! You are doing great. However, I am sure there are an equal number of us who are thinking, "I *know* what I am supposed to do. I am using visualization to create positive and negative food associations, which has helped a lot. I am meeting with my support team, celebrating our victories together. That has helped, too. Nevertheless, I still struggle to find time to cook healthy foods and avoid cookies."

This chapter is about two things. Mostly, it is about the specific diet system I use and recommend to patients aiming to lose weight. This system synthesizes many of the findings we have discussed in this book. It is designed to reduce inflammation, prevent insulin spikes, and manipulate calorie intake and fat metabolism as efficiently as possible to melt fat away.

However, this chapter is *also* about ease and convenience. It is about removing the *necessity* for motivation and willpower as much as possible and giving you options you feel great about instead of temptations to resist. This chapter focuses on intensely practical tips for making your eating plan easier rather than on any deep psychology of general motivation.

So, without further ado, here are some practical tips to make life easier for *anyone* adopting a new eating plan, no matter what eating plan that might be.

Make It Easy

There are a few basic steps we can take to make eating well as easy as possible for ourselves. These steps require planning. That is *all* they require; with proper advanced planning, they should not require large amounts of motivation, willpower, or effort. It would be best to think far enough ahead to make these choices effortless.

Control What You Buy

The first intensely practical tip is this: let laziness be your ally. I mean controlling what foods you keep in the house. The day it becomes marginally more convenient to eat an avocado than to bake or order or go out to buy cookies or cake is the day you will successfully eliminate those foods from your diet. Not having tempting foods in the house will almost completely remove the willpower component from avoiding them.

Of course, you want to make sure that you still have convenient, tasty, and satisfying options in the house. That is what the rest of this chapter will be about: making dishes that are as easy, healthy, and delicious as possible.

But let's be honest: not having cookies and cakes in the house will help a lot.

Take a moment to ask yourself: what are ten unhealthy foods you tend to overindulge in? Can you eliminate these from your shopping list in the near future? We will give you healthy, delicious foods to replace them with soon.

If even restraining yourself from putting cookies in your shopping cart sounds strenuous (believe me, I get it), try this: wait for a day when you're free in the morning and go grocery shopping first thing in the morning.

This really does work. You will be shocked by how little you desire Oreos and Little Debbies when you go shopping first thing in the morning. You may also be shocked to find how downright appetizing the produce section seems.

The temptation to buy unhealthy foods when we shop is a function of stress and fatigue. I know how hard it can be to restrain oneself from buying cookies because I have been there. At 6:30 pm, after a long day at the office, my self-discipline and decision-making capacities for the day were utterly exhausted. In the place of a well-rested, happy brain, I had stress hormones and fatigue signals circulating in my blood.

Not so at 6:30 *am*, when I am bright-eyed and bushy-tailed. First thing in the morning, I feel no temptation to add junk food to my cart and instead am happy to buy the items that I know will help me reach my health goals.

This is a well-established principle of diet science. However, I wanted you to know that it works for me, too.

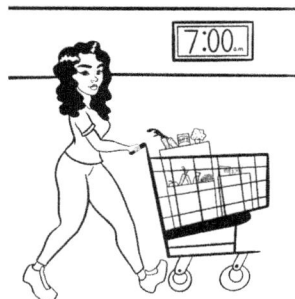

When we shop early in the morning, we have more willpower and fewer cravings.

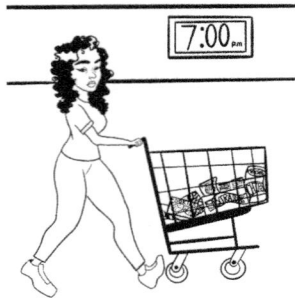

When we shop after a long
day, we have less willpower
left and more cravings for
junk food.

MAKE YOUR MEAL KITS

You may have noticed that I am *cooking* healthy and delicious foods. I am not talking about buying frozen or pre-prepared meals. That is because pre-prepared meals—even those sold by diet plans or "health food" companies—are often quite unhealthy. They may pile on the sugar and preservatives in the service of being low fat, or they may add highly processed saturated fats to meet the requirements of low-carb diets. Either way, they are not the *optimal* choice for health. Instead, it is much better to prepare your meals using fresh, whole ingredients from scratch.

How then, you might ask, can I also claim to be minimizing the effort you'll be required to put into this plan? The answer is called the "create your meal kit" approach.

As you may have noticed, "meal kits" in which a company sends you a box containing pre-measured portions of precisely the ingredients you need to make a recipe are all the rage. Kits like Hello Fresh and Blue Apron offer great healthy meal options as fun and straightforward as opening the box, slapping it all together in a pot or skillet according to the directions included in the box, and enjoying the results.

This approach almost eliminates preservatives and other secret, unnatural "taste enhancers" from the equation and allows you to maximize the natural deliciousness of fresh ingredients. If that is the best and easiest option to help you eat healthy, by all means, go for it.

However, there are a couple of problems with most meal kit services, which I also want to address here.

One is that paying people to do the labor of preparing and shipping those boxes is not cheap; you can expect to pay at least twice as much for a meal kit as you would to buy the ingredients yourself in bulk from the grocery store. For many families, that difference is a big deal.

This is why I will teach you how to put together your own meal kits by buying ingredients at the grocery store and preparing them yourself. This requires planning ahead regarding what meals you want to eat for the week and putting a couple of hours per week into prep work and shopping. However, if you do both of these things, you will have a week's worth of Blue Apron-worthy meal kits constructed with life-extending and fat-melting ingredients that are probably cheaper than the pre-prepared junk food you might have bought instead.

Steps to the "make your meal kit" lifestyle:

1. Procure a set of at least seven food storage containers large enough to store ingredients for a whole meal. These can be Tupperware, glass, or anything else that will fit in your fridge.
2. Also, procure seven or more freezer bags of the suitable size to store enough raw meat to feed your family for a single meal. If you live alone, this may be just a tiny Ziploc bag, while feeding a family of six may require a much larger container.
3. I say to procure at *least* seven containers because you may wish to prep to cook just one full meal per day, or you may want to cook from scratch for breakfast, lunch, *and* dinner. Some home chefs may also wish to store certain ingredients for the same recipes in separate containers to avoid premature flavor mingling.
4. Decide what you want to eat for each meal you plan to prepare this week. If you want to make things as simple as possible and do not mind repeats, you may choose just two

or three recipes to shop for; if you like variety and are cooking for more than one meal each day, you may choose up to 21.

5. If you choose to make many different recipes in a week, look for recipes with overlapping ingredients. The uses of oatmeal in breakfasts and desserts, for example, are nearly infinite. Oatmeal can be given many different textures and flavors when paired with different companion foods and a variety of cooking methods without requiring you to buy seven different base kinds of cereal for your breakfast and dessert plans.

6. Make a list of the ingredients you will need for each recipe, including the quantities of each. Multiply the quantities needed for each serving by the number of people you need to feed and the number of days you plan to eat this recipe this week.

7. Compile these into a master shopping list. If necessary or helpful, take another look for spots where the same ingredients could serve in more than one recipe to simplify and cut down on waste.

8. It is time to go shopping! When buying your ingredients for the week, consider how you will store perishable ingredients for the future.

9. When sauces or stir-fries call for fresh herbs that can only be bought in bulk, for example, I like to make "flavor cubes." Using an ice cube tray, I will mix a diced herb or a blend of diced herbs so that when I need this flavor combination in the future, I can throw an ice cube in the skillet. Just remember to label your ice cube trays if you do this to avoid getting an herbal surprise in a cold drink!

10. Once the ingredients are purchased, divide them into the storage containers you got earlier. Ingredients that are safe to eat raw such as fruits, vegetables, grains, eggs, etc., can be stored together in the refrigerated Tupperware; ingredients that are unsafe to eat raw and which may spoil if refrigerated for more than a few days, such as raw meat and

seafood, can be stored in the freezer bags you procured earlier.

11. When the time comes to cook each meal, pop open your self-made meal kit and assemble it according to the instructions in the recipes you found. If you choose your recipes expertly, this will take no more than half an hour to fresh, delicious, healthy food that you made yourself!

Now, if you have more money than time on your hands, ordering a pre-made meal kit from a company may be an easier way for you to accomplish this goal. Nevertheless, I did mention that there are two problems with many of those meal kits, and I want to talk about the second one now.

The meal kit companies are concerned about selling food that most people want to order. They are healthy enough to use fresh, raw, whole ingredients for the most part, but they are probably not optimized for people who are attempting rapid weight loss, rapid muscle gain, or a longevity-promoting diet. This is why learning to make your meal kits gives you additional power: you can have the convenience of a meal kit throughout the week, but with the precise foods chosen to optimize your health goals.

And with this in mind, we now come to the real meat of this chapter. I want to share the eating plan I have used for my weight loss, which combines many of the principles we have discussed in this book so far.

This eating plan uses three "phases," each designed to optimize the metabolism in different ways. Phase 1 is optimized for rapid weight loss, Phase 2 for gradual weight loss, and Phase 3 for weight maintenance while focusing on anti-inflammatory and longevity-promoting foods.

Dr. T's Eating Plan: Phase 1

The first phase of my eating plan is designed to radically change your hormone balance and cravings while rapidly dropping excess fat and water weight. This phase is designed to produce immediate results for the first thirty days of your fat loss journey but can be adhered to longer if desired.

In Phase 1, no sweeteners, caloric *or* non-caloric, are allowed. This is because sweet-tasting compounds, even if they are calorie-free, may still stimulate insulin spikes that can lead to fat gain and fat retention, as well as cravings for more sugar.

In Phase 1, carbohydrates of all sorts are severely limited. This is not because all carbs are bad, but because carbohydrates can spike insulin and can be high in calories. Carbohydrates acquired by eating fruits and green veggies are okay, but grains, most starchy root vegetables, beans, and sweeteners of any kind are off the table. Do not worry: healthy, nutrient-dense complex carbohydrates will be added back into your eating plan after one month, once your body's sugar cravings and insulin spikes have been tamed.

I also advise patients to stay away from dairy during Phase 1. There is evidence that many people have a low-level inflammatory response to dairy proteins in their bodies. This is different from lactose intolerance and is not acute enough to be considered an allergy by most health experts. However, experts on inflammation believe that low-level inflammatory responses to dairy might be a significant factor in feeling bad and aging prematurely.

The foods that are *recommended* during Phase 1 include:

- All the green vegetables you can eat. It is almost impossible to overeat when it comes to low-calorie, nutrient-dense superfoods like artichokes, asparagus, beets, peppers, broccoli, cauliflower, Brussels sprouts, cabbage, onions, carrots, parsnips, radishes, turnips, mushrooms, eggplant, squash, and salad greens of any kind.
- Fruit in moderation. I would not eat a whole watermelon, but two or three servings of fruit per day are high in fiber, vitamins, and minerals, while they may simultaneously help to satisfy any remaining sweet craving. To prevent a rapid blood sugar spike and crash, remember to eat fruit in the same meal as a lower-carb food, such as a salad or healthy fat.
- Nuts and seeds are a great source of heart-healthy fats, fiber, and proteins. Almonds, Brazil nuts, cashews, chestnuts, walnuts, hazelnuts, macadamia nuts, pine nuts, pistachios,

sunflower seeds, sesame seeds, and pumpkin seeds are among the healthiest. These nuts are high in calories, but their high-fat, low-carb composition means they will encourage fat burning in your cells.

- Of note, I do *not* include peanuts on this list because some evidence suggests that peanuts may make inflammation problems worse. I promise sun butter and almond butter are just as tasty and versatile for sandwiches and cooking as peanut butter!

- Other fats and oils. Avocado oil, walnut oil, olive oil, flaxseed oil, and canola oil are among the healthiest fats for your heart and brain. Despite officially being a fruit, Avocado is composed mainly of fat and can serve as an excellent substitute when a craving for creamy dairy fats strikes.

- Of note, flaxseed oil can impart flavor and nutrients to a dish, but it should *not* be heated. It can be added to soups and porridges after cooking but should not be added *before* cooking or reheating. When flaxseed oil is heated, its healthy fats rapidly break down into other types of fats which smell rancid and are bad for you.

- Egg whites are a great lean source of protein. I recommend keeping your egg yolk consumption down to one yolk per day due to the yolk's cholesterol content, but egg whites can be used to make omelets, frittatas, added to cobb salads, and much more.

- Lean meats in moderation. Lean beef, pork, and chicken breast are high in protein and specific vitamins and minerals. Fish and shellfish are also good additions to your eating plan. However, pregnant women should try not to eat more than a few servings of fish per week due to the hypersensitivity of developing fetuses to mercury and other nasty chemicals that fish may pick up in today's unfortunately polluted oceans.

How might you combine the elements listed above into delicious, nutritious meals during Phase 1? How might fresh fruit take the place of refined carbohydrates in your diet? What about replacing dairy fats with equally creamy avocado or healthy kinds of nut butter? What about roasting or boiling green vegetables instead of starchy roots for your side dishes? How about lean marinated chicken breasts instead of fatty burgers? You may be surprised by how flavorful a properly marinated chicken breast can be.

Consider meals like:

- Fruit and avocado smoothies with a teaspoon of flaxseed oil for added extra health benefits.
- Vegetarian or meat-based stir-fries and curries with lots of flavorful vegetables.
- Keto "burgers" feature deliciously marinated, grilled lean meats, flavorful veggie toppings, and crisp lettuce wraps. If cheese is sorely missed, a flavorful cheese sauce can be made from roasted, salted cashews soaked and blended in a food processor.
- Oven-roasted seasoned veggies or nuts in place of French fries or cookies. Once you have mastered your veggie seasoning game, you may never want to return to the old snack foods again.
- Snacks consisting of fresh fruit and nuts or nut butter for a delicious combination of the sweet and flavorful and the creamy and salty.

During this phase, you will want to make sure you eat *at least* 1200 calories per day. This is the lower limit of the recommended caloric restriction for longevity in adults. You will recall that advocates of fasting for longevity often placed their estimates at eating around 20% less than the standard baseline calorie consumption for an adult of your gender and body weight; none recommend eating less than 50% of your baseline caloric need for safety reasons.

Scientists now believe that 2,000 calories is a bit low for most adults in terms of basic caloric need; 2,400 is closer to a safe number to use to calculate the *minimum* caloric intake that a person should have.

Furthermore, 50% of 2,400 is, of course, 1,200 calories. This is the absolute minimum number of calories recommended for daily consumption to avoid the risk of serious complications such as the potentially lethal refeeding syndrome which can happen when someone who has had insufficient food intake for an extended period of time reintroduces calories to their diet suddenly.

I say to make sure you eat at *least* 1,200 calories because many of these foods are so filling and satisfying that people sometimes mistakenly stop short of this mark. For this reason, I do not believe you need to count calories to avoid overeating. Still, you will want to avoid eating too *little* to ensure you are getting enough calories to maintain a healthy metabolism.

There is a world of flavor and texture to be discovered among these ingredients. Do not let it go to waste.

DR. T'S EATING PLAN: PHASE 2

After a month or so of Phase 1, some people's bodies will begin to require more carbohydrates to function well. Phase 2 allows you to maintain fat loss and higher energy while permitting a more comprehensive array of foods than Phase 1.

During Phase 2, you can eat all of the foods from Phase 1, plus:

- One serving per day of unprocessed starchy food such as beans, potatoes, quinoa, pearled barley, bulgur, brown rice, steel-cut oats (no instant oats!), bread, or pasta. Ezekiel bread is an ideal bread option, as it is more nutrient-dense than other types of bread and so will give your body more than just calories.
- One serving per day of rice milk or almond milk. I suggest avoiding these in Phase 1 as they are likely to be highly processed and contain sweeteners unless you have made them at home yourself.

During Phase 2, enjoy your oatmeal, sandwich wraps, fruit-and-almond-milk smoothies, and the odd side of brown rice or whole-grain pasta. Remember to keep carbohydrates to about one serving per day and continue loading up on nutrient-rich veggies, fruits, and nuts.

Phase 2 can be maintained for as long as you wish to continue losing weight. It has the added benefit of being suitable for your blood sugar and energy levels due to the high nutrient density and the relative lack of insulin spikes which can cultivate insulin resistance in your cells. The slight decrease in the pace of your weight loss during Phase 2 will be accounted for by the presence of increased carbohydrates in this diet. Nevertheless, that is not wholly a bad thing: most people's bodies seem to work best when they have *some* carbohydrates in their diet in the long term.

As usual, ensure that you eat at least 1,200 calories per day. Interestingly, you will find it easier to unwittingly eat more calories now that insulin-releasing carbohydrates have been added back into your diet. For this reason, it is a good idea to continue to exercise discipline in your portions of carbohydrates. To keep things lean, consider meals like:

- A smoothie made of fruits and rice or almond milk.
- A cup of oatmeal with generous servings of sweet fruits and heart-healthy nuts mixed in.
- Delicious open-faced vegetarian or meat-based sandwiches served on a slice of grilled or toasted Ezekiel bread.
- Add a cup of brown rice to your stir fry for a little extra carbohydrate-based fuel.
- Add a cup of cooked barley to your veggie-based soup for more body and texture.

DR. T'S EATING PLAN: PHASE 3

Phase 3 is designed to be the maintenance phase. It is not intended to spur further weight loss but rather maintain your desired weight and energy levels without falling back into old habits that could encourage weight gain or blood sugar problems.

In Phase 3, all of the foods you have eaten during Phase 1 and Phase 2 are available to you. However, it is also time to add more culinary flexibility. I recommend using ONE of the following two options, according to which sounds better to you:

Add an additional daily serving of carbohydrates if you wish. That may or may not sound good to you at this point.

OR

Schedule one weekly "cheat meal." For this meal, eat whatever you want to enjoy a full range of life's culinary pleasures! Make this *only* one meal, not a full day of binge-eating, to avoid upsetting your hormonal balance and undoing months of progress. Moreover, remember to *enjoy* that meal. After all, we experience health problems not because certain foods are "evil" but because we become addicted to them and begin to eat them mindlessly without truly appreciating their culinary value.

It may be interesting to watch your cravings once you reach Phase 3 and compare those to the cravings you had when beginning Phase 1; you will likely find that, due to hormonal changes, many of the foods you once craved no longer sound nearly as appealing to you after a few months of practicing Phase 1 and 2 eating.

You can switch between Phases 1, 2, and 3 whenever you like. I do encourage everyone who reads this to try living by Phase 1 for at least one month to see the immediate benefits. However, after that month, some of you may reach your target weight, or you may begin to experience symptoms associated with a lack of carbohydrates. If so, moving on to Phase 2 is a good idea.

You can stay in Phase 2 for as long as you like. Furthermore, when you decide it is time to move on to Phase 3, you can do another month of Phase 1 or Phase 2 at any time to reap the benefits of revving up your metabolism and attuning your hormones.

I hope that the knowledge in this chapter will help you reach your health goals. Weight loss is a primary goal for many Americans, both for cosmetic and health reasons. Nevertheless, this eating plan is designed to do much *more* than help you lose weight. This eating plan promotes longevity and healthy aging, boosts energy levels, and prevents or even reverses harmful health conditions. To stay motivated on your eating plan journey, let us do a quick review of the benefits of using these three eating phases in your life:

- A nutrient-dense diet means more vitamins, minerals, and fiber. All of these are associated with better health outcomes in various health conditions. You will find yourself better-protected against the health risks of micronutrient deficiencies than most people in the developed world.
- Compared to the average modern diet, the low-carb nature of this eating plan helps you avoid insulin spikes, insulin resistance, diabetes, and weight gain. When paired with exercise, blood sugar levels and insulin resistance can significantly improve over time.
- The emphasis on heart- and brain-healthy fats in this diet, while excluding unhealthy, dangerous fats like those found in dairy, fatty meats, and processed foods, can reasonably be expected to convey protection against heart disease and other disorders stemming from atherosclerosis (hardening of the arteries due to fat and cholesterol build-up).
- The lack of refined carbohydrates, combined with micronutrient density, improves energy. Your mitochondria become more efficient at turning the food you eat and the air you breathe into energy when they are not swamped with glucose all the time. Every aspect of your metabolism functions better when supplied with adequate vitamins and minerals of all varieties.

Remember to *enjoy* this eating plan. It is not a diet; its goal is not to temporarily restrict your eating but to build a whole new lifestyle based around the healthiest (and tastiest) foods available. The limits of this diet are more than made up for in encouraging the creative use of nature's most juicy and flavorful ingredients.

The hardest part of this eating plan for many people is the time required to cook these meals from scratch since pre-prepared meals virtually never meet these health requirements. To that end, I hope that the ideas for "DIY meal kits" will help you to make this eating plan as convenient and affordable as possible.

I hope you have a fantastic journey to better health and superior cooking skills!

CHAPTER 10

MUSCLE MASS: YOUR SECRET ALLY IN WEIGHT LOSS

I have a deeply personal reason for encouraging my patients to maintain their muscle mass and strength, especially as they age. My mother fell victim to "sarcopenia"—muscle breakdown that doctors deemed a "normal" symptom of aging.

Independence was important to my mother. She always needed to be able to choose where she went and when. She wanted to do everything herself. This was true right up until she slipped one day while working in the kitchen, cracking her pelvis.

For doctors, a broken hip like this is a grave omen: broken hips have high rates of complications and are often harbingers of fatal blood clots and infections.

Although I knew these dangers, I was optimistic when my mother was admitted into the hospital. She was an otherwise healthy older woman, and it seemed sure that surgery would have her back on her feet in no time.

Tragically, this is not what happened. After her surgery, my mother began experiencing chest pain and shortness of breath. Because she had been treated for panic attacks with anxiety medication for most of her life, both my mother and her hospital nurses mistook this chest pain for symptoms of a panic attack.

In reality, she was suffering from a massive pulmonary embolism—a blood clot that blocks arteries in the lungs, destroying the body's ability to move oxygen into the blood. These embolisms are more common after certain types of surgery, disrupting blood vessels deep in the body and causing clots to form. Surgery to repair a broken hip is one such procedure. My mother's broken pelvis killed her, and sarcopenia is to blame.

Muscle mass loss is an important cause of falls that result in broken bones for the elderly.[1] In recent years, the link between falls and tragic, early death in older patients has become so well-known that fall prevention has, in turn, become a number one priority for doctors in several disciplines, as well as in medical and elder care facilities.[2] The fewer accidental falls a facility sees, the fewer patients die tragically sooner than they need to.

As we all get older, our bodies create less muscle mass and less strength after engaging in the same amount of exercise. Suppose we lead sedentary lifestyles as most Americans do. In that case, this can lead to a severe loss of strength and ultimately problems with balance, which is dependent on the strength of muscles all over our bodies to keep us precariously balanced upright on two legs.

In my mother's case, her advanced age made her more prone to falling and more prone to sustaining a broken bone since bone density and strength also decline with age. Once she fell and fractured her hip, she was at risk for many complications, including the one that ultimately killed her.

The thought that my mother may have lived years or decades longer if she had been more physically fit still haunts me. At the time of her fall, no one in my family prioritized exercise or physical fitness for our elderly relatives. They were not athletes, after all, even in their youth. What would they do with a few extra pounds of muscle mass or impressive athletic abilities for their age?

After my mother's death, my way of thinking changed.

What if we all developed programs to gain muscle mass in our youth and maintain our athletic physique into our old age? What if we did this, not as a means to an arbitrary end like a sporting competition, but as a means to stay alive?

LOSS OF MUSCLE MASS

Although sarcopenia has been accepted as "normal" and therefore inevitable and untreatable by many mainstream medical authorities, the truth is that sarcopenia is entirely preventable. With the correct exercises and diet choices, it is even entirely reversible.[3]

When people in the modern world approach losing weight, they often think almost entirely about calories in and calories out. Weight loss and building muscle are often two separate, unrelated, and perhaps even contradictory goals. Bodybuilders speak of "bulking up," while weight loss programs speak of "slimming down." The two would appear to be mutually exclusive. However, the opposite is true.

When calories are deficient, the body—surprise—cuts its energy expenditures. This means that the fewer calories you eat, the fewer calories you burn. This is likely part of *why* caloric restriction seems to improve health and lifespan; the body simply cuts back on its exertion, resulting in reduced wear and tear. Nevertheless, it also means that losing weight through calorie restriction alone is much harder to do than most people realize. That is why, in this book, we will explore two critical additional components of weight loss. Moreover, one of these is building muscle.

You may have heard that muscle burns more calories than fat at rest. Our bodies contain a gene that explicitly inhibits muscle growth because, if this function is not inhibited, the muscle we build through everyday activity will consume so many calories that it would risk fatally starving our brain under natural conditions.

A little boy named Liam Hoekstra was born without a working copy of the gene for myostatin—a protein whose name means "to stop muscles." From an early age, his parents noticed he was ripped. By the time he started elementary school, little Liam had six-pack abs, rippling biceps, and the ability to perform feats of strength that stunned surrounding adults.

Fortunately for Liam, he was born in a developed nation after the industrial revolution; his parents could feed him a special, ultra-high-calorie diet to ensure that his brain did not suffer due to all the calories his muscles consumed. Without access to this diet, Liam's remarkable muscle mass may have caused him life-threatening medical problems.[4]

The point is that muscles burn calories. They are also lovely for various reasons, including increased physical strength, increased balance and ability to resist injury, increased energy and vitality, and cosmetic appeal.

If you are an older reader, you may have been told that you are losing muscle mass, and you can do nothing about it. This is untrue. Although losing muscle mass and strength is one of the "symptoms of aging" that most medical authorities have long considered "normal," there is nothing inevitable or irreversible about it.

"Sarcopenia" is a term for loss of muscle mass and strength. It comes from the terms "sarco" for "muscle" and "penia" for "want or lack of." When it happens to young people because of illness or an injury that prevents them from using their muscles, "sarcopenia" is considered a disease symptom that needs to be treated. However, when it happens to us as we get older, it is considered "normal" and is often not addressed with any treatment regimen.[5]

This is a shame since sarcopenia is preventable and reversible in people with normal, healthy muscle-building genes. All that is required to treat and reverse sarcopenia is to perform the proper exercises to build strength evenly across the body.

At the end of this chapter, I will share some of these exercises with you. However, first, let us take some time to examine why sarcopenia occurs as we get older and how these exercises work to combat it.

THE STRANGE TRUTH ABOUT MUSCLE GROWTH

In the realm of science fiction and fantasy, super strength is a much-desired trait. Sometimes it is achieved through scientific advances, such as a super-soldier serum or a genetic mutation. However, the truth is almost the opposite.

It is not that it is *difficult* for our bodies to make muscle. We contain a mechanism to restrain the runaway freight train that is our natural muscle growth capability. Instead, the problem is that muscle tissue absorbs so many calories that our body refuses to build more muscle than is needed, lest we accidentally starve ourselves.

Our ancestors had to worry about starvation and malnutrition *a lot*. That is why our bodies would rather store fat than build muscle and why even our very bones will wither away if we do not use them. When we are not using a bone or muscle regularly, we effectively tell our body that we do not need it to survive. So, to save on energy and nutrients, our body obliges by actively breaking down our "unneeded" bones and muscles. The only tissue that *does* not disappear if we do not use it is fat because fat is there to *protect* us against starvation conditions our body is so worried about.

So how can we tell our bodies that we need those muscles? By using them, of course. We can say to our bodies that we need *more* muscle by exercising the muscles we already have to the point of exhaustion, sending our bodies the simple message that we need more muscle to deal with the heavy physical demands of our existence.

Most bodies in the developed world are not *required* to perform heavy physical labor. Most of us pay our bills sitting down, and the absolute most strenuous jobs have us performing repetitive movements in a factory or warehouse. These repetitive movements can cause more health problems than they solve since they neglect most of the muscles in our body while placing a repetitive strain on just a few muscles and joints. Paradoxically, an excellent full-body exercise routine can *improve* the overworked warehouse staffer by building a more substantial base of whole-body muscles and bones to support our overtaxed areas.

Several things contribute to the slowdown of new muscle production as we age. Our cells, including stem cells, gradually accumulate DNA damage, making it just a little harder for them to produce healthy new cells. Our hormone levels change, giving our bodies the idea that we are no longer in the prime of our reproductive health, and we may not *need* that extra bone or muscle so much. Now, our bodies are more likely to "choose" to conserve energy and calories rather than build themselves up to perform feats of endurance.

Note the phrasing there: "more likely." It does not become impossible to build new muscle, or even bone mass, as we get older. It takes more time and effort to get the same level of performance than a younger person. This slowing of the rate at which our bodies produce new tissues in response to exercise, combined with modern sedentary life of older people, has caused many doctors to give up on preventing or reversing age-related muscle loss. Many doctors feel their patients are unlikely to do their prescribed exercises or do not see any acute need to prevent or reverse sarcopenia since most of their patients are not professional athletes or models.

To get ourselves to actually perform strenuous physical exercise regularly, we have to be self-motivated. Unless we are professional athletes, performers, or soldiers, our jobs will not reward us for working out every day. With no *necessity* to do so, it is easy to simply *not* do it at all.

Because the significant obstacle to unlocking this secret to weight loss and health is our habits, let us take this opportunity to revisit some of the cognitive tricks we learned to teach ourselves in order to enjoy activities we might have previously grown to dislike.

If you have not yet implemented the suggestions from previous chapters, you may wish to revisit the end of Chapter 1 to see my complete list of tips and tricks to change your habits and love every minute.

A list of the easiest "hacks" to support your exercise routine includes:

- Exercise in the morning, when you have more energy and are more likely to make healthy choices. This will allow you to start your day already feeling great about what you have achieved.
- Find the type of exercise that *feels* best to you. Does vinyasa yoga make you feel much better than hitting the gym? Do you love to run outdoors on a beautiful day with a great playlist or audiobook in your ear? Can you watch your favorite movie or TV show while you are on that treadmill or exercise bike?
- Find role models of your own demographic to inspire you and to compete against. I know many elderly people who had an "if she can do that, why can't I?" moment when a

video of Ruth Bader Ginsburg's fitness routine went viral during her treatment for pancreatic cancer.

- Whatever your age, body type, or ethnic background, I can promise you will find people like yourself performing inspiring feats of athletic prowess on YouTube and other online platforms.
- Level up. By creating fitness and exercise goals and then hitting them, you can "gamify" your exercise experience and get excited about hitting the next milestone.

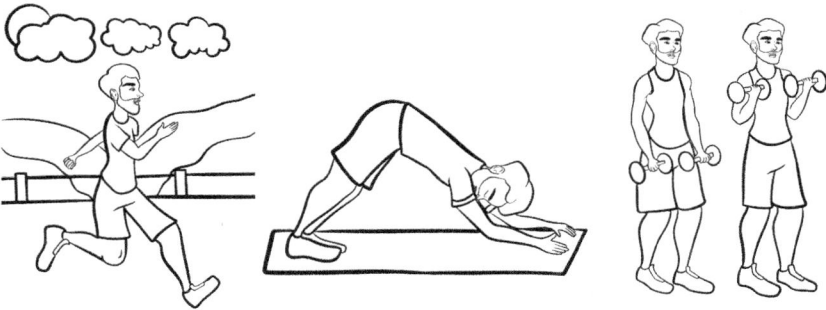

There are many different ways to reap the metabolic and cosmetic benefits of exercise.

Doctors are currently divided about when, and whether, to diagnose sarcopenia in patients with low muscle strength or age-related muscle loss. Recognizing the dangers of muscle loss and weakness, sarcopenia is now designated an official disease in the ICD-10 diagnostic coding system used by doctors.

However, critics point out that there is no general agreement about exactly *how* weak someone's muscles or how rapidly their muscle deterioration must be to qualify as sarcopenia. There is also no good evidence to suggest that diagnosing sarcopenia as a disease leads to improved outcomes, since doctors generally encourage people to exercise and strengthen their muscles regardless of age or diagnosis.

Some doctors fear that health insurance and pharmaceutical companies may take advantage of increased sarcopenia diagnoses to increase patients' insurance rates or to prescribe pharmaceuticals that may not be helpful and could potentially do harm. For this reason, the same patient may be diagnosed with sarcopenia, or *not* diagnosed with sarcopenia, simply depending on which doctor they happen to visit.[6]

Know that muscle strengthening is virtually always good for you, so long as you are not damaging other body parts like your joints in the process. The stronger you build your muscles early in life, and the more active you remain later in life, the less likely you will be to fall victim to tragic accidents like the one that killed my mother.

If a doctor tells you that you have sarcopenia, that's a strong indicator that your health could be at serious risk if you don't exercise more to cultivate muscle strength, balance, and control. But even if you are not diagnosed with it, remember that maintaining a healthy level of activity and muscle mass is not just aesthetically pleasing: it can be life-saving.

CHAPTER 11

HEALTH & FITNESS HACKS: VIBRATION TECHNOLOGY

Many fitness gurus have amassed fortunes promising fitness "hacks," which allegedly allow exercisers to build more muscle mass using less time and effort. These have ranged from the fraudulent to the scientifically sound. Some include options that carry extreme health hazards or even six-figure price tags.

Elaborate machines have been created that use cold water, blood pressure cuffs, extreme weight loading, and other techniques to improve metabolic gains from relatively fast and easy exercise routines. Some of these may be advertised as "must-haves" for those serious about fitness. However, one much more accessible technology has tested better than most of these contraptions: the vibrating platform.

In vibration therapy, subjects may perform exercises, lie down, or stand on a vibrating platform. These platforms appear to significantly improve health and fitness gains for the amount of time and energy put into the exercises. As with all exercise equipment, vibration therapy may not be necessary for a healthy person who is highly successful at exercising using traditional methods. Nevertheless, vibration technology shows promise for people who may struggle with exercise and health gains due to conditions like obesity or sarcopenia.

Once, the reason vibration technology worked seemed obvious:

being subjected to hundreds of vibrations per second would cause the body to automatically engage in hundreds of muscle activations to compensate for the movement. This would effectively turn the simple act of standing on a vibrating platform into exercise - an exercise that did not require much conscious exertion to perform and which could work the muscles to exhaustion in a short amount of time.

Lately it has become apparent that more is going on here. Vibration therapy has been shown to improve strength, bone mineral density, balance, and stability. [1] It has also been found to speed up fat loss potential.[2] This makes vibration technology a promising ally for those struggling to accomplish health goals, especially healthy older people for whom questions of bone mineral density, balance, and stability may be particularly urgent.

How does vibration technology accomplish all of this? At this point, no one is sure. Some hypotheses are still examining the neuromuscular activation performed by the body in response to vibration. However, it is unclear if these responses would be able to generate the wide-ranging results seen in vibration therapy.

Clinical studies suggest that the best results are achieved when patients use vibrating platforms for 12 weeks. Vertical vibration platforms appear to yield better results than horizontally oscillating platforms. The best results were obtained from whole-body vibration techniques in which the entire body experiences some vibration. Platforms with larger vibration amplitudes–those that move more with each vibration–showed more substantial gains than those with slower-amplitude vibrations.

Scientists reviewing clinical trials of vibration therapy gains also found that performing a combination of isometric and dynamic exercises on the vibrating platform led to the most significant benefits.

Isometric exercises test the muscles without the movement of joints. Examples of isometric exercises include planks and wall sits. The theory is that simply activating muscles without movement should strengthen these muscles for the future. While this does have some effectiveness, more significant gains are usually seen from dynamic exercises, which work out multiple muscles because they involve taking the body through a range of motion.

Dynamic exercises involve the movement of joints: these are exercises such as squatting, lifting weights, or doing sit-ups or push-ups. These can carry more risk of injury because pressure is placed on a joint in motion. However, the exerciser also benefits by working a more comprehensive range of muscles and exerting more force.

Vibration research scientists recommend that people first use isometric exercises, which offer more stability and lower risk of injury when becoming accustomed to a vibrating platform or other vibrating equipment. To gain maximum benefit, dynamic exercises can be introduced over time as the exerciser becomes more stable and accustomed to the vibrating equipment.

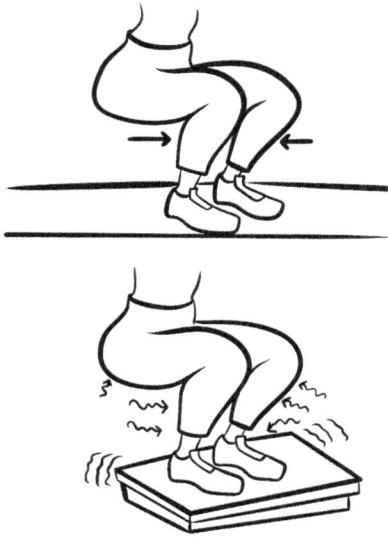

Scientists are not sure why vibration conveys benefits for strength training, but it may have to do with more nerve and muscle activation.

Because exercising on a vibrating platform can be so physically intense, the best results seem to occur when exercise is broken up into 30 to 60-second sets with about a minute of rest in between for a total vibrating workout time of about 15 minutes per session.[3]

You can see this technology's time and energy efficiency appeal; the best workouts took 15 minutes per day, with only up to half that amount of time spent exercising. That is something that even the busiest or most exercise-averse patient is likely to be able to accomplish.

The benefits of whole-body vibration training go well beyond reaching fitness goals. In a literature review conducted by a different team of scientists, it was found that whole-body vibration training may assist with weight loss. It also had other, more mysterious metabolic benefits. Authors Zago et al. found that vibration training for at least six weeks improved the body's ability to regulate blood pressure and reduced artery stiffness, a significant risk factor for heart disease and stroke. Vibration training for more than ten weeks resulted in significant decreases in body weight and improvements in blood sugar regulation and insulin resistance in obese women.

No one quite knows how full-body vibration training accomplishes some of these effects. Scientists are speculating on the mechanism, but more data is needed to confirm whether these theories are correct or if something completely different is at work. To date, the leading hypotheses are that nerve stimulation through vibration may have action deep inside the tissues; that blood sugar and insulin improvements may be related to the muscle work performed during vibrating exercise; and that the release of growth-related hormones, thought to be due to the effects of vibration training on muscles, may lead to these body-wide effects.[4]

The combination of fitness and health outcomes from whole-body vibration training makes this an appealing addition to any exercise or health improvement routine. Although scientists are still seeking more data about *why* whole-body vibration therapy does so much, there is solid evidence to suggest that the benefits are significant.

As with all medical treatments or exercise routines, there may be contraindications for the use of vibration technology. Some users have complained about joint and muscle pain.[5] These appear most commonly among significantly older adults with very advanced sarcopenia, certain obese patients whose joints may be strained by their body weight, and people with connective tissue disorders resulting in fragile joints or muscles.

However, vibration technology has been used safely and effectively in older adults with mild to moderate sarcopenia and in overweight people to improve some of the significant health concerns that come with these medical conditions.

While you may not need a vibrating platform for your home if you are succeeding well with conventional exercise techniques, it may be worth talking to your doctor about using a vibrating platform, particularly if you or a loved one is struggling to make gains in essential areas of health and safety. Those with acute concerns about bone mass density, balance, stability, and obesity may benefit the most.

Caution is needed to avoid falls and other injuries that can result from losing one's balance or overuse. The good news is that vibration technology may allow you to "hack" your workout without breaking the bank. Of course, proper use and supervision is a must.

CHAPTER 12

THE TRUTH ABOUT WEIGHT LOSS

Now is an excellent time to get into the granddaddy myth of weight loss —the axiom that eating fewer calories sheds pounds, as does burning more calories through exercise. As Colonel Potter used to say on *M*A*S*H*: horse hockey!

Losing weight is not so much about eating *less*. If you only cut your calorie intake and don't change the kinds of foods you're eating, studies show that your body will adjust its metabolic rate down and simply burn fewer calories.[1] Weight loss is much more about eating *differently*.

The same goes for exercise. Exercise does not help you lose weight at the rate of some simple formula of calories burned equals pounds melted off. Exercise *will* help you lose weight and enjoy better health in every aspect of your life, but it is not as straightforward as reality TV shows and gym advertisements would have you believe.

Let us start with food and how our bodies use calories. By understanding the *truth* behind weight gain and weight loss, we can lose weight far more efficiently (and pleasantly!) based on the best experimental data we have available. We need no longer rely on calorie counting and other restrictive diets.

This is not about "one magic food" or anything like that. Instead, it is about understanding what makes us feel full, what stimulates cravings, and why so many of us put on pounds every year. The following chapter will also cover how our bodies respond to exercise from a calorie-burning standpoint, which is probably far weirder than you have ever imagined.

Earlier, we mentioned Dr. Jason Fung's finding that insulin—a hormone released in huge quantities by our bodies when we eat refined carbohydrates—makes us fat. Insulin effectively tells cells to store all those delicious carbohydrates as fat. Whether we are getting it by eating carbohydrates or injecting it therapeutically, the result is usually the same: get the dosage just a tiny bit too high and weight gain results.

However, it turns out that this is only part of the story. For the rest of the story, we must turn to Dr. Herman Pontzer. An associate professor of evolutionary anthropology and global health at Duke University, Dr. Pontzer has probably done the most impressively thorough assessment of how human bodies burn calories of anyone in history.

Moreover, the results are *profoundly* bizarre.

Dr. Pontzer uses a method called "doubly-labeled water" to very precisely determine how many calories of food any given animal has burned to make energy in a given day. This is quite a remarkable and challenging feat. Scientists had been estimating how many calories they thought a given activity *should* burn based on very rough measurements taken under questionable laboratory conditions.

It turns out that everything you have ever heard about calories is hilariously wrong. The average adult does not burn 2,000 calories per day or less, and our bodies do not *keep* burning 2,000 calories per day when we starve ourselves. You probably did not burn 600 extra calories with that hour of yoga yesterday.

Nevertheless—here is the crucial part—that hour of yoga probably made you much healthier, and likely to live longer, in some exciting ways. Furthermore, you *can* convince your body to lose weight by changing your diet. But you cannot usually do it simply by eating fewer calories. Successful weight loss typically involves minimizing or eliminating foods which cause insulin spikes; intermittent fasting to get your body into fat-burning mode; and increased exercise to build muscle mass.

To learn the details of precisely how doubly-labeled water allows scientists to measure *precisely* how much fuel a given animal has turned into energy recently, I highly recommend Dr. Pontzer's excellent book *Burn: New Research Blows the Lid Off How We Burn Calories, Lose Weight, and Stay Healthy.*

For now, let us say it is awe-inspiring. Here are the basics:

Dr. Pontzer's research first gained notoriety when he did an exhaustive analysis of how many calories were burned by the hunter-gatherer Hadza people of Africa. A typical Hadza adult walks for miles each day and spends a good chunk of their time climbing trees, digging in the hard-packed dirt of the African savanna with wooden sticks, and performing other feats of athleticism and endurance that would challenge the average American athlete.

Conventional wisdom suggested that the Hadza must burn far more calories than the average American. Based on the crude estimates used by many "calories burned" estimation apps, the average Hadza adult should burn *thousands* more calories per day than the average American adult. When Dr. Pontzer's exhaustive study of the Hadza showed that they *did not*, the collective jaws of the entire metabolic medicine community dropped.

The Hadza did not just burn fewer calories than expected. They burned almost precisely the same number of calories as the average sedentary American burns sitting on their couch.[2]

What in God's name was going on here?

The thing is that this actually makes perfect evolutionary sense. Life would be twice as difficult for the Hadza, who work so hard for their food if they burn twice as many calories as we do every day. That would not work very well.

However, this reality also means that our bodies are much weirder than we ever imagined. At a deep level, the Hadza's cells are working entirely differently from those of a sedentary American to allow them to hike miles, climb trees, and spend hours on labor we might consider backbreaking without burning more calories than we do.

Dr. Pontzer's new data described a world where the human body burns roughly the same amount of calories, no matter its activity level. There are exceptions to this—research has shown that genuinely extreme athletes who engage in full days of strenuous exercise *can* burn far more—but as far as levels of activity that our bodies can sustain in the long-term without dying, they all burn pretty much the same amount of calories.

Now, the important thing is that bodies with different activity levels *spend calories on different tasks.* This turns out to be why exercise helps us feel better and live longer: our bodies become drastically less healthy, including craving more food and carbohydrates, when we do not exercise. Nevertheless, this is not because exercise is burning calories that we would not be burning; exercise burns calories that would otherwise be spent on potentially harmful biological processes like inflammation.[3]

We will cover more of how exercise takes calories *away* from harmful body processes, extending our lives and helping us make healthier choices in the next chapter. Let us focus here on what *not* to do when seeking to lose weight and what works.

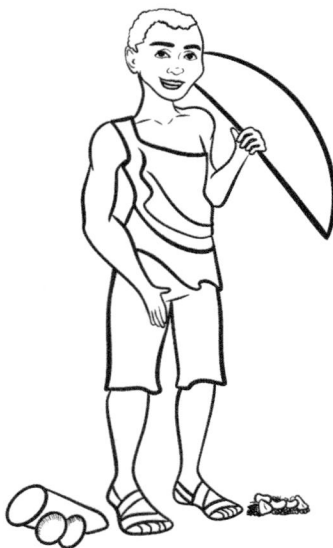

Hadza hunter gatherers do eat carbohydrates, but they are unrefined carbs such as root vegetables, wild seeds, and honey. This is probably how many of our ancestors ate.

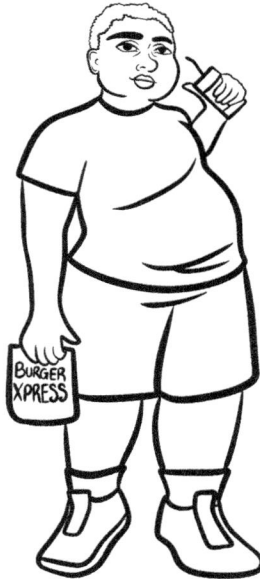

Many modern diets include lots of
refined carbohydrates such as
sugar and white flour. These cause
our bodies to store fat, and can
cause many health problems
because of their metabolic effects.

HOW TO BURN FEWER CALORIES

Note that the heading above is not "how to eat fewer calories." I will not tell you to eat fewer calories because that almost certainly would not help you lose weight. Nevertheless, learning how your body might *burn* fewer calories is essential.

Remember, burning fewer calories can slow your weight loss or cause you to *gain* weight by storing fuel as fat instead of burning it as energy. And what is a pretty good way to make your body start *burning fewer calories*? It is simple: you *eat fewer calories*. This is why caloric restriction is not a very good weight loss tool: it is just as likely to cause your body to cut back on calories burned, leading to future weight gain, as it is to cause your body to burn fat.

This, too, makes evolutionary sense. If you have less food available, your body pretty much *has* to find a way to get by on fewer calories. Furthermore, we know it is capable of doing this: after all, if the Hadza can get by on barely more than 2,000 calories per day, you can probably live on half that.

The problem, of course, is that this makes it much harder to lose weight. It leads to "rebound" weight gain seen in many people who lose weight primarily through calorie restriction.

Of course, extreme calorie restriction *does* cause short-term weight loss. However, it can result in *long-term* reductions in the number of calories your body burns. By starving your body, you have successfully sent the message that it needs to burn fewer calories and store more energy as fat for the subsequent inevitable famine.

When you then return to eating a "normal" amount of calories after you are satisfied with your weight loss (or you have given up because the diet is too unpleasant), your body may store *more* of that food as fat than it did before you started while burning less when you exercise. This is anything but a desirable outcome.

It is interesting to note that there is one circumstance under which long-term caloric restriction *may* have desirable effects. This is the caloric restriction diet situation, which David Sinclair has cited as a powerful life extension tool.[4]

When we combine Sinclair's research with Pontzer's, an exciting possibility emerges. Pontzer's research suggests that exercise conveys its benefits by diverting calories from potentially destructive processes like inflammation to more beneficial ones like muscle growth. Is it possible that the caloric restriction diets function on the same principle?

By eating 20-30% fewer calories than its species would typically consume, the animal test subjects and human proponents of caloric restriction for life extension may effectively accomplish the same effect as burning 20-30% of a normal-calorie diet through exercise. 20-30% of calories are lost to reproductive processes and overzealous immune responses in both cases. Just as Sinclair predicts, Pontzer's research shows that humans divert energy away from reproductive functions and toward long-term survival when food is scarce. Sufficient exercise may also cause our bodies to divert energy away from non-essential body functions.

If you want to use caloric restriction for its health benefits, cutting your calorie intake to 70-80% of your normal levels is not a bad strategy.

However, if you plan to eventually start eating normally without counting calories again, using a calorie restriction diet may make you heavier in the long run.

If that sounds like a recipe for disappointment, what can we do instead?

HOW TO LOSE WEIGHT

Dr. Pontzer's findings in Hadza communities raised some obvious questions. If humans burn roughly the same amount of calories no matter how much they exercise—or don't—why are so many of us fat?

Dr. Fung's work in *The Obesity Code* suggests one apparent reason: refined carbohydrates are strongly correlated with weight gain, at least in part through their roles in unnaturally spiking your insulin levels. There is also far more to the story than that.

Dr. Pontzer goes out of his way to debunk the Paleo Diet idea that hunter-gatherers ate no carbohydrates at all. He points out that *most* known hunter-gatherer cultures get *most* of their calories from carbohydrates. Data to the contrary is based on some dubious-at-best extrapolations from preliminary 20th-century reports, and this "low-carb paleo" idea is directly contradicted by more rigorous hands-on studies of living hunter-gatherer peoples today. [5]

However, the carbohydrates eaten by the Hadza are very different from those eaten by most Americans. The Hadza get their carbohydrates primarily from wild-foraged, undomesticated yam-like root vegetables, from wild ancestors of modern grains, and honey.

Do you recognize those recommendations from anywhere? If you said, "sweet potatoes, whole grains, and honey are all carbohydrates recommended to promote weight loss and prevent diabetes," you are right! These natural carbohydrates, which have *not* been through thousands of years of selective breeding and industrial refinement, have radically different effects on our insulin than modern refined carbohydrates.

As a result, they are "safe" for weight loss, while white sugar, white flour, white potatoes, and white rice can play havoc with our metabolisms.

Dr. Fung attributes most of the weight-gain qualities of refined carbohydrates simply to their ability to spike insulin. This is undoubtedly accurate, especially given that even artificially administered insulin causes weight gain. Dr. Pontzer uncovered another exciting pattern.

Modern, industrialized humans may be gaining weight because our diets are too delicious.

Pontzer and Fung both share the observation that it is actually not easy for a human to gain weight rapidly. Even intentional gainers often struggle to put on more than a few pounds per month. [6] [7]

This is yet more evidence for the idea that the human body tries as hard as it can to maintain caloric equilibrium: it will do its best to maintain your weight right where your hormones say it should be, regardless of how much or how little you eat. Your body thinks this is how it helps you to survive, regardless of whether your problem is famine or an overabundance of Twinkies.

However, our body *does* appear to have an error rate of a few percent when it comes to overeating. These small percentage points can result in putting on a few pounds per month or per year. This is particularly true if the food we eat is high in refined carbs, which cause insulin spikes that the body may interpret as a signal that it is *supposed* to store more fat.

Now, what about the behavioral angle of weight loss?

As it turns out, studies of eating behavior show that people eating highly processed foods tend to eat more calories. This is not just because highly processed foods tend to *have* more calories; people eating foods high in refined carbs, salt, and fats will eat a larger quantity of food than people eating fruits, vegetables, and lean protein. This is one more way that refined carbohydrates and processed foods drive weight gain.

One reason for this might be immediately apparent to you: those processed foods sound way more delicious than the natural, healthy alternatives I mentioned. Moreover, this deliciousness may overwhelm your brain and your hormone system. If food is sufficiently tasty, you may continue eating long after your body begins sending "cease and desist" signals in the form of satiety hormones and a full stomach.

That is how you gain weight, despite your body's best efforts to prevent you from doing so. Unfortunately, this is also behavior that is now culturally accepted and even socially rewarded in modern American culture. Processed foods take less time and effort to prepare. In many cases, they may even be cheaper because the ungodly amount of chemicals in them gives them a long shelf life and makes them less expensive than fresh food to transport.

As Dr. Pontzer so astutely points out in *Burn*, this is no accident. Food companies employ whole research divisions of food scientists with the specific goal of making their food as *addictive* as possible.

This is how they make money, and is one reason why many scientists advocate for stricter regulations on these companies and stricter labeling laws. Some of those food scientists saw the current epidemics of obesity and diabetes coming decades ago by looking at the trend of steadily more addictive foods entering the marketplace. Unfortunately, those food scientists who spoke up were largely unsuccessful at getting companies to use healthier ingredients and labeling practices.[8]

Fortunately, there is only so much you can do to make a raw fruit or a fresh vegetable addictive. Lean cuts of meat will probably never reach potato chip levels of "you cannot eat just one." That is a perfect thing for our survival.

That is why, in this book, we are concentrating on easy, nutrient-dense made-from-scratch meals. Our goal is to provide food that will nourish you correctly even if you choose to do some caloric restriction for the health benefits and help you lose weight *even if you do not*.

How does that work?

The foods mentioned above also have several other important characteristics which they share with their healthy whole-grain cousins. These traits will help you naturally eat less because your body will signal that food is plentiful *without* getting a weight-gain-inducing insulin spike. Over time, this can cause your body to "decide" that your optimal weight is lower than your current weight due to the reduced levels of insulin signaling.

These characteristics shared by whole grains, fruits, vegetables, and lean meats include:

1. Fiber. Do you know how whole grains are darker in color and crunchier than refined carbohydrates? A lot of that is sweet, sweet fiber. It takes up space in our guts, setting off "stretch receptors" that tell our brains when we have eaten enough. Fiber also feeds the bacteria in our guts that improve our health and prevent colon cancer. Legumes, vegetables, and fruits are also stuffed full of fiber.

2. Protein. Those fibrous bits of whole grains also include bonus protein. Even fruits and vegetables are high in protein relative to refined carbohydrates. Moreover, meat, of course, is made of the stuff. Protein also helps us to feel complete. When specific sensors in our guts detect protein, they send additional "we have eaten enough" now signals to our brains.

3. Healthy fats. Fats can also send "we have eaten enough" signals to our brains. However, be careful: saturated fats such as animal fats are *also* very delicious. If our food is delicious enough, we may ignore our "I am full" signals and keep eating. That is one reason why vegetable fats are generally healthier than animal fats. Vegetable fats also tend to contain fatty acids that are *good* for our hearts, while the fatty acids in animal fats are often harmful to them.[9]

These ingredients also have another thing in common: none of them are found in refined carbohydrates.

To summarize: for weight loss and health, choose foods high in fiber, lean protein, and plant fats; avoid refined "white" carbohydrates like the plague to keep your insulin responses under control.

This is what it means to eat like a hunter-gatherer. Eat like this, and your body will soon restore itself to a healthy equilibrium in terms of weight *and* other important markers of health, well-being, and longevity.

CHAPTER 13

THE TRUTH ABOUT EXERCISE

The most surprising truth about exercise is one we mentioned in the last chapter. Exercise *does* burn calories—but unless you are spending a full day at the limits of human endurance, it does not do it in a way that will directly cause weight loss.

Barring the most extreme (and dangerous, unsustainable) exercise routines, exercise does not increase the total number of calories we burn per day. Instead, the calories we burn through exercise are *deducted* from other bodily functions, such as our immune and reproductive functions.

That sounds bad, right? We want our immune system to have all the energy it can get. We want our reproductive systems to be functioning correctly.

Or do we?

WHAT'S GOING ON WITH HUMANS AND EXERCISE?

Dr. Pontzer explores the metabolic differences between humans and chimpanzees. Although they are our closest living cousins, human and chimp metabolisms are shockingly different. While chimpanzees burn far fewer calories per day than humans and can stay perfectly healthy lazing around in zoos all day, humans burn far more calories, and being lazy seems to kill us.[1]

At first sight, this is pretty bizarre. While many doctors of human medicine assume that diseases that plague us, such as heart disease, diabetes, obesity, and arteriosclerosis, are inevitable results of primate laziness—simply what happens when we allow our bodies to atrophy— Dr. Pontzer's findings suggest something else.

Chimpanzees do not get human-style heart disease. Their arteries do not harden with age. They do not gain weight and maintain fat reserves comparable to those of the leanest human athletes, no matter how much food you give them or how little time they are given to move around. Chimpanzees never die of clogged arteries or diabetes: they die of other things. This is true even when they burn far fewer calories and exercise far less than an average human.

What mechanism would explain all of these observations? Why should our closest cousins be designed to be so much more efficient, while humans burn through our food reserves at an alarming rate, yet still manage to get fat if we eat processed foods and die if we do not perform an amount of exercise that a chimp would regard as crazy?

Dr. Pontzer suggests that the answer lies in the behavioral changes that have allowed us to have big brains.

Humans, as it turns out, are spectacularly weird among the primate family. All other great apes burn drastically fewer calories than we do. None of them seem to need exercise to stay healthy or alive. None of them get fat when they overeat. None of them are bipedal. Furthermore, none of them hunt large game as a major part of their diets.

Dr. Pontzer suggests that all of these differences may be related to one core survival strategy.

Humans are what zoologists refer to as "persistence hunters." We do not think of ourselves as elite athletes in the animal world because we cannot sprint as fast as a cheetah or a deer, but we can run much *farther*.

Indeed, it is considered a reasonable proposition to chase down and kill a cheetah among African hunter-gatherers. It is not that hard: the cheetah may sprint at 60 to 70 miles per hour, but it can only do so for a small fraction of a mile. After that, the cheetah will have to stop to rest.[2] As anyone who has run a marathon can tell you, the human chasing the cheetah will not.

Humans, then, are superior runners compared to cheetahs. In fact, over a distance of miles, we are superior runners to *any* other animal. We may well be the only land animal on the planet that can run a marathon.

Why is that, and what dreadful consequences does it have for our metabolism?

I mentioned earlier that persistent running would kill cheetahs at an alarming rate. After just a fraction of a mile, a cheetah's lungs cannot move oxygen into its blood fast enough to feed its brain, and its muscles begin to overheat. Doing this a few times without stopping to eat a tasty carcass will exhaust the animal's resources so thoroughly that there is a good chance it will die before it can catch a life-sustaining meal, even if it is not intercepted by the spear of some patient persistence hunter who has been following it all this time at a slower pace.

Cheetahs and humans have one crucial thing in common: we are both hunters. The consequences of this for *Homo sapiens* cannot be overstated: even though meat makes up a relatively tiny portion of the hunter-gatherer diet, it's high in protein and fat, which makes it an invaluable resource for growing big brains.

It is also possible that this analysis overestimates the importance of hunting while underestimating the importance of intense physical activity in *Homo sapiens*-style gathering. I want to make sure we note this because there has, admittedly, been something of a male chauvinist bias when discussing the relative contributions of hunting and gathering to human development.

While hunting is said by many to be the most critical trait allowing humans the necessary protein intake to support our massive, world-dominating genius brains, it is just as possible that *cooking* is even more critical. Cooking food, it turns out, makes protein and other nutrients from all sources much more bioavailable, effectively increasing our nutritional intake by leaps and bounds.

EVOLUTION

There is no organ more demanding of nutrition than the brain. In the human fossil record, the invention of cooking occurs around the same time that the human brain begins to rapidly grow larger. From this, many scientists have suggested that cooking in fact *enabled* the development of our big brains by providing the nutrition that such massive minds demanded.[3]

Moreover, meat makes up a relatively tiny percentage of the diets of most hunter-gatherers. Neither is it the only human food-getting adaptation that is athletically intense: the vast majority of hunter-gatherer calories come from *gathered* foods, with the two primary sources for Dr. Pontzer's Hadza being tubers and honey.

Now, here is the thing about tubers and honey: they do not run away from you, requiring a marathon to chase them down, but they *do* require intense athletic activity to obtain.

For hunter-gatherers, digging up tubers requires hours spent digging in hard-packed earth with just a stick. Obtaining honey usually involves climbing trees—the most athletically and calorically intense activity we measured, in part because it is often completed with the aid of tools requiring intense physical exertion, such as the use of hammers to drive stakes into trees to create a makeshift ladder in order to reach otherwise inaccessible beehives.

Like persistence hunting and running marathons, these gathering techniques are athletically and calorically intense activities that no other animal engages in. This is *why* these feats of athleticism serve the Hadza so well: no other animal uses sticks to dig otherwise inaccessible tubers out of the ground or routinely climbs trees to break open bees' nests to get honey.

So it may be that the importance of being "persistence hunters" has been drastically overblown. In contrast, the importance of cooking and tool-use gathering may be drastically underappreciated.

Either way, the result is the same: humans have enjoyed such explosive success as a species because we rely on calorically expensive methods of procuring food. Like the cheetah's 60-miles-per-hour sprint, our method of feeding ourselves is metabolically expensive. However, just like the cheetah, our expensive skills make us *the best in the world* at procuring these types of food, whether we are referring to meat or naturally occurring carbs.

This may well have fueled the shift in human evolution to burning more calories on a routine basis than any other great ape. If we could expend several times more calories than our chimp cousins on gathering and hunting daily, we would need more food daily. Nevertheless, we would also *get more* food to support massive brains capable of advanced teamwork and advanced technology.

With that advantage, no other species on the planet stood a chance of out-competing us, even if it meant we needed to eat like the chimpanzee equivalent of Michael Phelps during training season.

The problem is that our big brains may have done their jobs a little too well for our good. What happens when a species designed to burn massive amounts of calories through physical activity each day stops doing that?

Cheetahs are designed to run. They are specialized to be so good at it and rely on it so heavily as a survival strategy that the metabolic side effects and the number of resources they pour into running will kill them if they do not use their gift as nature intended.

Now, what if humans are similar? What if we are designed so exquisitely to run and hunt that *not* running kills us?

Cheetahs risk dying of excess body heat and metabolic depletion if they run for too long. Humans appear to risk dying of arteriosclerosis and high blood sugar if they *fail* to run for too long.

The principles at work in both cases are shockingly similar: in both cases, the body is doing something that will prove fatal if we do not adhere to our evolved survival strategy. The body deems this an appropriate trade-off because this survival strategy works incredibly well, making us top predators and top innovators.

What adaptations might we expect our bodies to undertake over a million or so years of our ancestors burning 500+ calories exercising every day? Furthermore, why might our bodies evolve this bizarre "caloric constancy," where they burn just as many calories at rest as they do while active, so long as adequate food to support this is available?

Let us revisit Dr. Sinclair's theory regarding the survival vs. reproductive pathways within cells. In Dr. Sinclair's assessment, when resources are scarce (such as during times of extreme dietary caloric restriction), cells focus on staying alive to survive until more great times come along before reproducing.

When a time of plenty *does* arrive in Sinclair's model, cells turn their attention toward reproduction. This activity is good for the propagation of the gene pool but costly and risky for the individual. An activity that, in Dr. Sinclair's theory, leads to accelerated aging.[4]

This is not to suggest that you should not have kids: but it is worth noting that being in reproductive mode *all the time* may be costly. In "Burn," Dr. Pontzer observes that Hadza women only have a baby about every three years, despite a lack of birth control.

This is because the caloric costs of Hadza daily activity suppress reproductive function in both men and women, diverting calories away from the sex organs and resulting in lower levels of circulating sex hormones. Hadza women ovulate less, and Hadza men produce less sperm. Pontzer notes humorously at one point that sedentary American men may expect that ripped Hadza hunters who routinely steal the game from lions have more testosterone than them. However, the reverse is true.[5]

I do not believe that sex hormones are a primary cause of aging or heart disease. As we have discussed earlier, they can stave off some signs of aging when boosted naturally. However, I wanted to discuss them because they are one obvious, easily measurable indicator of non-essential body processes being repressed by caloric restriction, whether it be from a caloric restriction diet or engaging in the levels of exercise that nature intended for us.

Now again, "suppressing non-essential bodily functions" probably sounds terrible. Nevertheless, what if it is not? What if our bodies have evolved to *over-express* certain bodily functions during periods when not burning 500 calories per day gathering food?

This would make sense. All available research suggests that when calories are scarce relative to caloric needs, the bodies of *all* animals prioritize essential over non-essential metabolic tasks in order to stay alive. Suppose you belong to a species whose athletically intense lifestyle leaves you in a state of relative caloric scarcity almost all the time. Wouldn't it make sense to adapt to that restriction by keeping most processes suppressed most of the time and then turning them way up to compensate when the opportunity arises?

Instead of sex hormones, let us take a moment to look at immune function. Immune function consumes a lot of calories. Enough that it is suppressed during "fight or flight" states in order to free up calories and energy for the essential function of running away from lions, as we discussed when talking about the role of cortisol earlier in this book.

Now, we might think that having lots of calories available for the immune system to do its job is a good thing. It *is* if you are acutely sick or injured. Indeed, that is another reason this mechanism would have made sense for our ancestors. If a Hadza became too sick or injured to hunt and gather, that person would suddenly have 500+ additional calories per day available for their body's immune and healing functions. Again, taking a few days without strenuous exercise as a metabolic cue to kick things into overdrive would have made sense.

However, what happens when things are in overdrive all the time? Could too *much* immune system activity, sustained over months or years, actually kill us?

OUR IMMUNE SYSTEMS AND INFLAMMATION

The skyrocketing number of individuals with crippling and life-threatening autoimmune diseases would say "yes." So would many doctors.

Inflammation has been called the most important marker of aging, or perhaps even the most important cause of aging, by many doctors who are interested in longevity. Inflammation appears to cause damage to practically every tissue in the human body as we age, and the kicker is that no one knows why this happens.[6]

Hardened arteries that lead to heart attacks and strokes, for example, are caused in part by high cholesterol as a result of eating unnatural diets. However, the *other* root cause is inflammation, a systemic immune response that damages tissues and whose root cause is poorly understood.

At its best, inflammation kills pathogens that might otherwise threaten to kill us. It is healthy and normal to have an acute inflammatory response for a couple of days after getting an acute injury or infection. Nevertheless, when inflammatory responses continue for weeks, months, or years, our tissues take nearly as much damage as any hostile invaders that get caught up in the response.

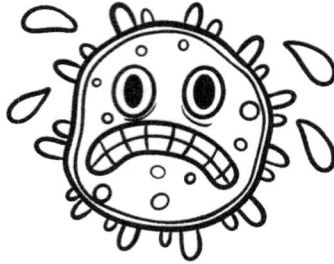

Cells that experience inflammation become stressed and damaged.

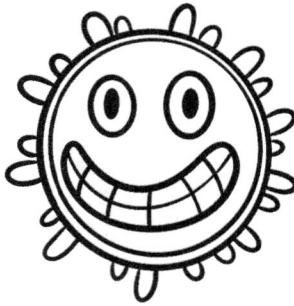

Cells function better when they aren't experiencing inflammation.

What if this excess inflammation happens because our bodies believe our sedentary lifestyles can only indicate that we are fighting a raging infection? What if the *reason* this only happens in humans, not in other great apes, is that our bodies have evolved to turn the heat up on infections—and on our tissues as an unpleasant side effect—whenever we stop moving for too long? Moreover, what if our bodies turn inflammation up directly to the amount of metabolic fuel we give them?

The results of experimental studies seem to indicate that this might be true. We know that:

- Eating refined carbohydrates increases systemic inflammation and risk of death from inflammatory diseases.[7] No one knows why this occurs.
- Aerobic exercise reduces systemic inflammation across the board. No one knows why this occurs.[8]
- Caloric restriction diets *also* reduce systemic inflammation and the corresponding tissue damage and signs of aging.[9]

It sure looks like our bodies produce damaging levels of inflammation in direct proportion to the amount of fuel we put into them that *is not* consumed by exercise.

Now, I also am not arguing that inflammation is *the* primary cause of aging or sedentary diseases. We know enough to know that there are still probably many processes operating in our bodies, regulating our health, which we have not yet even identified or begun to study.

However, if both reproductive and immune activity is suppressed by exercise—and this keeps us healthier—what other processes might be beneficial during short periods of rest but are harmful to us if we lead sedentary lives combined with a plentiful food supply?

It increasingly looks like the evolutionary adaptation of humans is not the Hadza's ability to burn no more calories than us when they spend their days hiking and climbing trees, but rather our own bodies' ability to keep burning Hadza levels of calories by ramping up our basal metabolic activity in the absence of exercise. Moreover, like the cheetah's adaptation to extreme speed, our adaptations may actively kill us when not used as nature intended.

There is no aspect of human health that is not improved by exercise. Scientists do not fully understand why that is. This new model, whereby our bodies begin to *actively* (if unwittingly) kill us when we spend too long being sedentary, may close the gap between several lines of evidence related to exercise, caloric restriction, inflammation, and primate metabolism.

Do not let this section get you down: after all, your body is not doing anything today that it was not doing yesterday.

Instead, use this knowledge as motivation to get up and move around, as a hunter-gatherer would!

CHAPTER 14

THE SPIRITUALITY OF HEALTH AND WEIGHT LOSS

The Bible says your body is a temple. To be exact, it states:

> *"Or do you not know that your body is a temple of the Holy Spirit within you, whom you have from God? You are not your own, for you were bought with a price. So glorify God in your body."*
> —*1 Corinthians 6:19-20 (ESV)*[1]

This brings a new dimension to the health and weight loss journey. While God probably does not care if we are swimsuit models or bodybuilders, one who believes in God likely also believes that God put us on Earth for certain reasons. And to carry out those reasons, we need a healthy vessel.

It is not just Christianity which teaches this. Indeed, religions around the world have treated physical bodies as gifts from our Creator, which we have the responsibility of stewarding well. From the disciplines of yoga, martial arts, and Chinese medicine which teach that physical and spiritual well-being and fortitude are innately linked, to exhortations to eat godly diets and avoid situations which may contaminate us with disease, religions and spiritualities around the world teach that our bodies have cosmic or divine significance.

Nor is this idea necessarily restricted to a theistic worldview. After all, religious people are not the only people who feel that there are many missions for us to accomplish in this world. Whether one's sense of purpose comes from honoring God or from alleviating suffering or accomplishing another goal in this world, chances are that accomplishing your purpose will be greatly helped by maintaining your brain and body in good working order.

For me, the parallel between my religion and spirituality and my health and weight loss journey is obvious. During Lent and on certain other holy days each year, the Catholic Church requires its followers to abstain from eating outside of three daily meals. Curiously enough, this bears a great resemblance to the intermittent fasting plan which is one of the most important components of my own routine for a healthy weight.

This parallel is so obvious that the priest at my local church has been known to make a joking disclaimer when announcing fasting days: "We're not doing this to lose weight." In fact, the stated purpose of this fast is to show and cultivate religious devotion through discipline, proving to ourselves and to God that we are willing to resist temptation for His greater purpose.

Now, you may or may not believe that the Christian God is the source of your greater purpose. But you probably do believe that you have such a purpose. If you don't, I might recommend getting that looked at: there are countless problems to be solved in the world, and countless things to be experienced. There is no shortage of purposes available to you, and studies show that people who feel that their lives are purpose-driven do better on major measures of mental and physical health.

Whatever your purpose in life is, it is reasonable to assume that having a healthy brain and body will make you more likely to accomplish it successfully. And, like it or not, that means eating and exercising well. You will likely struggle if you don't eat and exercise in ways that give you the mental clarity and physical ability to perform the daily tasks required for your purpose.

If you are a believer in a higher power, this relationship between yourself and the body you have been given takes on new meaning. After all, in a created universe there are no accidents; you were not placed here by the mere random movement of particles, but by a consciousness with loving purpose. And your body is not a mere accident of chance, either. It is a gift given to you for a specific purpose.

Of course, not everyone can have excellent physical health. Many theologians would argue that those with disabilities or chronic diseases were given those for a reason, too, possibly to facilitate spiritual growth. But we can all agree that doing what we can to maintain a basic level of health is helpful to whatever work we were sent into the world to do.

Now, hearing all this talk of "life purpose" might have one of two effects on you. One is the effect of empowering and motivating, giving a greater sense of importance to your own life and potential. The other is a sense of burden and exasperation; perhaps you don't need *more* responsibilities. Both responses are quite natural.

But let's discuss, for a moment, how one's sense of purpose is not the whole story when it comes to the spirituality of weight loss. What can the spiritual worldviews teach us about *how* to live healthy lives each day?

Your Spiritual Quest

Religious traditions don't embark on fasting, or on challenging physical endeavors, in order to lose weight or build physical strength. So why do they prescribe activities such as physical disciplines and special diets and eating schedules, if not to accomplish health or cosmetic goals?

Well, it's not about the physical outcome of the practice; it's about the experience of *doing* the practice.

Religious fasts are not intended to produce weight loss. They *are* intended to develop discipline and promote certain mental states. In the mindset of religious fasting, the difficulty of not eating between meals is not an inconvenience to be masked and forgotten as effectively as possible; that difficulty is the *point*.

The purpose of a religious fast is to demonstrate devotion and cultivate discipline by doing something difficult. The difficulty is not a mere side effect of a desired end goal: it is the whole purpose of the exercise. How much easier, then, must it be for the religious who fast to keep to their strict requirements compared to the fad dieters who see no inherent value in suffering for a cause or proving one's strength in the face of temptation?

I am not advocating starving yourself here; indeed, *anorexia mirabilis*, a dangerous excess of religious fasting, is a diagnosis listed right alongside *anorexia nervosa* in the handbook of medical diagnoses.[2] But for those who struggle to adhere to a healthy, doctor-approved intermittent fasting regimen in the service of mental clarity and weight loss, perhaps this mindset can reframe your struggle.

The same can be said of exercise as a spiritual pursuit. Religious seekers do not practice yoga, martial arts, manual labor or undertake long pilgrimages on foot because they want to look ripped or win a heavyweight championship. They do it because the practice of the physical art itself is a spiritual experience for them. To them, undertaking a task of extreme difficulty and dedication is in itself a spiritual experience. When they "feel the burn," it is a communion with their maker and a sign of their dedication to the purpose for which they were created.

In modern Western society, we tend to be fixated on physical objects and long-term outcomes. When undertaking any new practice, we ask "what will we get out of it in the end?" That's not a bad question: it is certainly *one* of the right questions to ask when deciding what activities will give you a good return on your investment.

Yet this question is also clearly not *enough*. The end result of a lifestyle of healthy diet and exercise is almost unbelievable: these practices can yield years or decades of healthy life, enhanced physical and mental abilities, physical beauty, and reduced vulnerability of illness and injury.

It is rumored that Robert Butler of the National Institute on Aging once said, "If you could package the benefits of exercise and a healthy diet into a pill, it would be the most widely prescribed medicine." (Though interestingly I could not find a primary source documenting him saying this.)

The promises of exercise are indeed near-miraculous, yet these scientifically validated promised payoffs are not enough to get most Americans to make these investments.

Clearly, then, focusing on our desired final outcome is not adequate. Perhaps we must take a page from the religious and spiritual people of the world and focus on the journey instead of the destination.

When every burn from a pushup or sore muscle or running an extra mile is experienced as an act of devotion to your life purpose, it becomes much easier to exercise. When every healthy meal and resisted temptation is experienced as proof of your discipline and determination, it becomes much easier to diet successfully. When the struggle *becomes* the reward, anything is possible.

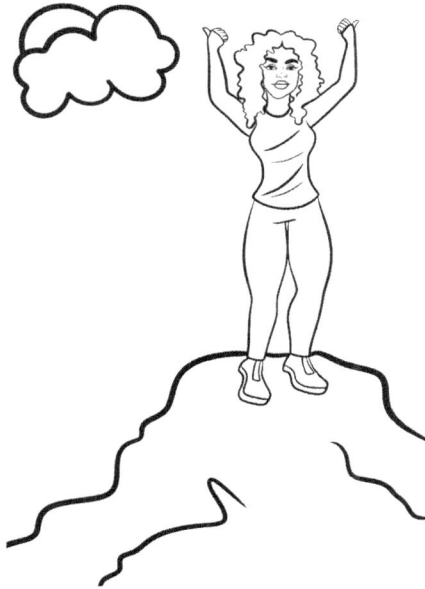

CHAPTER 15

YOUR TRANSFORMATION

We have now covered many tools that you can use to aid your journey of transformation. Remember that this transformation encompasses not only your appearance, but your health, your longevity, and the expression of your genes.

Stories like Jim's have shown us that there is no transformation that is beyond our reach; no matter how convinced you may be that you can never accomplish a goal, or that you simply "don't have the genes for it," you are overwhelmingly likely to be mistaken. Even family histories can't be a reliable indicator of our potential because our genetic source code can be overlaid by epigenetic programming. This programming can be changed in our lifetimes, resulting in radically different outcomes from those of our parents' generation.

If there is one thing I want you to take away from this book, it is this: this programming can be changed. When it comes to your body and your mind, very little is set in stone. You are your own to create.

I would urge my readers to remember to go about your transformation in a healthy way. It is no secret that even weight loss and fitness can be taken to unhealthy extremes, especially when we focus primarily on cosmetic changes while neglecting matters of deep health.

We may believe that we will see faster cosmetic results if we focus exclusively on our cosmetic goals; but the reality is that great, long-lasting cosmetic results come from the same processes that yield good organ health and an increased lifespan. For this reason, I urge you to focus on deep health such as stress reduction practices, nutritional and healthy eating, intermittent fasting, and whole-body fitness over some more popular approaches in cosmetic circles such as simple caloric restriction, fad diets, or workouts that exclusively emphasize cosmetic results to the exclusion of strengthening muscles across the body in a balanced way that enhances health and safety.

It is my hope that the information shared here will shape more than just your weight loss transformation. The principles of visualization, meditation, decision fatigue, good nutrition, stress reduction, and spiritual pursuits can transform every area of your life. Whether your goals include enhanced well-being, career enhancement, enhanced relationship, or enhanced creativity, these tools can make it easier to make the right decisions.

I am honored to have been a part of your journey of transformation. It is my belief that the work we undertake to shape ourselves, our lives, and the way we interact with the world is the most important work we can do. They say that change starts from within, with just a single person.

They also say that a journey of a thousand miles begins with a single step, and that is just as true. Every journey, no matter how epic, is made up of individual single steps which seem small and ordinary on their own. So when you feel discouraged, remember: just keep taking steps. Your steps are no less magical and powerful than those of the heroes you look up to.

What steps toward your goals will you take today?

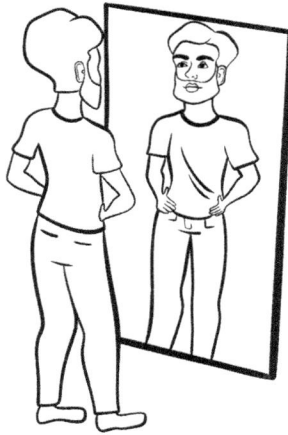

About the Author

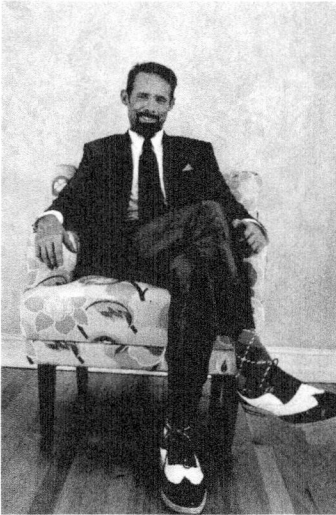

Dr. Francisco Torres is the author of seven books, including Keep Kicking Frisco, Keep Kicking, and Dr. T's Drop the Fat Cookbook. He has appeared on KevinMD and writes regularly for Doximity OpMed. He is a physiatrist in Clearwater, FL. He is affiliated with multiple hospitals in the area, including Largo Medical Center, Mease Countryside Hospital, Morton Plant Hospital, Tampa Community Hospital, and Morton Plant North Bay Hospital.

Dr. Torres received his medical degree from the University of Puerto Rico School of Medicine and has been in practice for 31 years. He speaks multiple languages, including Spanish. He specializes in pain medicine and sports medicine (non-surgical) and is experienced in physical medicine and rehabilitation, pain management, electrodiagnostic testing, musculoskeletal disorders, and age management.

When he's not treating patients or writing, Dr. Torres enjoys playing the violin and taking long walks on the beach with his dog, Gaudete. He hopes his books will help patients in the same way he has been helped by his numerous teachers and life experiences across the decades.

https://floridaspineinstituteandwellness.com/

Glossary of Terms

Acetylation—A method used by our cells to turn gene expression up or down. Acetylation can be thought of as a sort of "dimmer switch" on our genes, which can cause a given gene to be used more or less. We can alter the acetylation of our genes, and thereby how often our cells use them, through our lifestyle choices such as eating choices, stress management, trauma healing, and exercise.

Age management—The idea that the aging process, or at least many of its unpleasant side effects, can be slowed. Doctors and scientists who specialize in age management look for ways to help our bodies to continue functioning in peak condition for as long as possible through methods such as diet, exercise, supplementation, and medication. The use of medications to prevent signs of aging is controversial because the benefits and risks of doing this are not well-studied in humans.

Chromosome—A giant conglomeration of spooled-up DNA. Chromosomes are made of many histones, much like a giant collection of yarn made out of many smaller individual spools of yarn.

Downregulation—The "dimming" of a gene. When a gene is downregulated, it is expressed less often because biochemical changes in the cell have "told" the cell that that gene is not currently useful. We can send our cells biochemical messages to turn down less desirable genes through our lifestyle choices such as eating, exercise, trauma healing, and sleep. Every lifestyle choice we make changes the biochemistry of our blood in some way and making the right choices can lead to our desired gene expression outcomes.

Gene expression—The process of "reading" the information contained in your DNA and using it to build biochemical machines. What component parts each cell of your body is made of, and how that cell behaves, is determined by which genes are expressed in its nucleus. Biochemical changes sent to our cells change their gene expression. We can literally change what our cells are made of.

Histone—A structure used to organize DNA, similar to organizing yarn by wrapping it around a spool. Histones can also regulate which genes are expressed by winding our DNA tighter or looser, allowing transcription enzymes more or less access to genes. When DNA is spooled more tightly, it is less accessible and the genes within it are expressed less. When DNA around the histone is loosened, more copies of the gene can be made, and more of the cellular machinery it codes for can be produced. By sending biochemical messages to our cells to change their histone winding, we can change the component parts our cells produce. This is best accomplished through lifestyle choices such as eating choices, exercise, trauma healing, and stress management.

Insulin—A hormone which tells our cells to take in sugar from our blood and store it as fat. Insulin is released within our bodies in large quantities when we eat refined carbohydrates such as sugar and white flour. Over time, these large releases of insulin can lead to significant weight gain, and worse, insulin resistance. In the condition of insulin resistance, our cells stop responding to insulin because they have seen too much of it. Instead of taking sugar in, insulin-resistant cells allow sugar to remain in the blood, causing high blood sugar. Ultimately insulin resistance leads to the life-shortening disease called Type II diabetes. We can avoid or even reverse insulin resistance by strictly limiting our intake of sugar and white flour, and by exercising, thereby forcing our cells to use sugar from our blood as fuel for our activities.

Methylation—A biochemical process which turns genes "on" or "off." When a cell receives biochemical signals suggesting that a gene is not useful at this time, it can send enzymes to attach methyl groups to the DNA within the gene. These methyl groups block transcription enzymes from the gene, which means that the gene can't be expressed. Our bodies can turn genes on or off in response to personal or ancestral trauma, trauma healing, stress management, eating choices, and exercise. Trauma healing activities such as certain types of psychotherapy have been shown to change DNA methylation in patients with ancestral and personal trauma.

Longevity—The length of our lifespan is called "longevity." When people refer to longevity-promoting treatments or lifestyle choices, they are referring to activities which are intended to lengthen one's lifespan. Some "longevity-promoting" activities and medications have not been well-tested, but others, like healthy eating choices and exercise, are known to make significant positive differences to lifespan in most people. A tiny percentage of the population appears to have genes which cause extreme long life almost regardless of lifestyle choices, but unless most of your grandparents lived past 100, you are likely not among that tiny percent!

mRNA—mRNA, or "messenger RNA," refers to the RNA copies of DNA information which are used by cellular machinery to make the component parts of your cells. The "master blueprint," DNA, never leaves the protective membrane of the nucleus because cells are designed to protect their DNA at all costs. Instead, copies of the genetic information are made out of RNA and disseminated throughout the cell to workstations which "read" the instructions. The basis of mRNA vaccines is the injection of human-made mRNA directly into your cells to give them instructions that help them recognize viruses. This process cannot change your DNA, because mRNA copies cannot be reverse transcribed into DNA.

NMN—Short for "nicotinamide mononucleotide," NMN is a bioactive chemical which is promoted by scientist David Sinclair as a longevity-promoting supplement. Although NMN has shown very strong results in energy levels and life extension in laboratory mice, almost no data on the effectiveness of NMN in humans exists as of this writing. As of early 2022, only a few tiny studies on the effects of NMN on people or human tissues in petri dishes had been conducted. Nonetheless, it is worth noting that NMN studies did appear to show some improvement of metabolic health and slowing age-related tissue damage.

Sarcopenia—Harmful loss of muscle mass and strength. Sarcopenia can occur as a result of certain diseases and injuries, but always occurs as a result of advancing age if healthy levels of exercise are not maintained. In fact, doctors are currently debating to what extent it is possible to prevent or reverse sarcopenia in old age by using exercise. They are also debating how severe the loss of strength and muscle mass needs to be before sarcopenia is classified as a medical problem and not just a normal sign of aging. Muscle loss can be prevented through exercise at any age, although patients who already have severe muscle loss may struggle to recover through exercise.

Sirtuins—Proteins involved in the maintenance of DNA which David Sinclair believes to be involved in the aging process. Sinclair theorizes that aging occurs when DNA becomes damaged and cannot be repaired due to inadequate availability of sirtuins. Sinclair believes that his experiments on mice and yeast show that age-related damage to DNA can be prevented, or even reversed, using dietary and lifestyle choices. Sinclair also advocates for the use of medications and supplements such as NMN, though very little data exists about whether NMN has the same health-enhancing and life-extending effects in humans as it has in laboratory mice.

NOTES

1. ACTIVATE YOUR GENES, CHANGE YOUR LIFE

1. Klein, Jan; Klein, Norman (2013). *Solitude of a Humble Genius - Gregor Johann Mendel. Volume 1, Formative years.* Berlin: Springer. pp. 91–103. ISBN 978-3-642-35254-6. OCLC 857364787.
2. National Institutes of Health. (n.d.). *The discovery of the double helix, 1951-1953 | Francis CRICK - profiles in science.* U.S. National Library of Medicine. https://profiles.nlm.nih.gov/spotlight/sc/feature/doublehelix.
3. *Diploid.* Genome.gov. (n.d.). Retrieved June 22, 2022, from https://www.genome.gov/genetics-glossary/Diploid#:~:text=Diploid%20is%20a%20term%20that,cells%20contain%2023%20chromosomes%20pairs.
4. *Why is genetic diversity important?* Genetic diversity & evolution. Retrieved June 22, 2022, from http://maize.teacherfriendlyguide.org/index.php/genetic-diversity-and-evolution#:~:text=Genetic%20diversity%20is%20important%20because,providing%20the%20flexibility%20to%20adapt.
5. U.S. National Library of Medicine. (n.d.). *What is a gene?: Medlineplus Genetics.* MedlinePlus. Retrieved June 22, 2022, from https://medlineplus.gov/genetics/understanding/basics/gene/#:~:text=A%20gene%20is%20the%20basic,more%20than%202%20million%20bases.
6. Khan Academy. (n.d.). *Transcription: An overview of DNA transcription (article).* Khan Academy. Retrieved June 22, 2022, from https://www.khanacademy.org/science/ap-biology/gene-expression-and-regulation/transcription-and-rna-processing/a/overview-of-transcription#:~:text=Transcription%20is%20the%20first%20step,DNA%20s-trand%20as%20a%20template).
7. Centers for Disease Control and Prevention. (2022, May 18). *What is epigenetics?* Centers for Disease Control and Prevention. Retrieved June 22, 2022, from https://www.cdc.gov/genomics/disease/epigenetics.htm#:~:text=Epigenetics%20is%20the%20study%20of,body%20reads%20a%20DNA%20sequence.
8. *Understanding the stress response.* Harvard Health. (2020, July 6). Retrieved June 22, 2022, from https://www.health.harvard.edu/staying-healthy/understanding-the-stress-response#:~:text=This%20combination%20of%20reactions%20to,quickly%20to%20life%2Dthreatening%20situations.
9. Public Broadcasting Service. (n.d.). *Can trauma be passed to the next generation through DNA?* PBS. https://www.pbs.org/newshour/extra/daily-videos/can-trauma-be-passed-to-next-generation-through-dna/.

2. OBESITY, PAIN, AND TRANSFORMATION

1. Demeulemeester, F., de Punder, K., van Heijningen, M., & van Doesburg, F. (2021). Obesity as a risk factor for severe COVID-19 and complications: A Review. *Cells, 10*(4), 933. https://doi.org/10.3390/cells10040933

2. Larsson UE. Influence of weight loss on pain, perceived disability and observed functional limitations in obese women. *Int J Obes Relat Metab Disord. 2004;28*(2):269–277.

3. Felson DT, Zhang Y, Anthony JM, Naimark A, Anderson JJ. Weight loss reduces the risk for symptomatic knee osteoarthritis in women. The Framingham Study. *Ann Intern Med. 1992;*116(7):535–539.

4. Okifuj, A.i & Hare, B. D. The Association Between Chronic Pain and Obesity (2015). *Journal of Pain Research, 8,* 399-408

5. Stone AA, Broderick JE. Obesity and pain are associated in the United States. Obesity (Silver Spring). 2012;20(7):1491–1495.

6. McVinnie, D. S. (2013). Obesity and Pain. *British Journal of Pain, 7*(4), 163-170.

7. *Ibid*

8. McVinnie, D. S. (2013). Obesity and Pain. *British Journal of Pain, 7*(4), 163-170.

3. DNA Regulation

1. National Human Genome Research Institute. (n.d.). *Human genome project faq.* Genome.gov. https://www.genome.gov/human-genome-project/Completion-FAQ.

2. Cox M, Nelson DR, Lehninger AL (2005). *Lehninger Principles of Biochemistry.* San Francisco: W.H. Freeman. ISBN 978-0-7167-4339-2.

3. Berger SL. Histone modifications in transcriptional regulation. Curr Opin Genet Dev. 2002 Apr; 12(2):142-8. doi: 10.1016/s0959-437x(02)00279-4. PMID: 11893486.

4. Perera BPU, Svoboda L, Dolinoy DC. Genomic Tools for Environmental Epigenetics and Implications for Public Health. Curr Opin Toxicol. 2019 Dec;18:27-33. doi: 10.1016/j.cotox.2019.02.008. Epub 2019 Mar 8. PMID: 31763499; PMCID: PMC6874218.

5. A., R. V. E., Martienssen, R. A., & Riggs, A. D. (2009). *Epigenetic mechanisms of gene regulation.* Cold Spring Harbor Laboratory Press.

6. Kristensen, L. S., Nielsen, H. M., & Hansen, L. L. (2009). Epigenetics and cancer treatment. *European Journal of Pharmacology, 625*(1-3), 131–142. https://doi.org/10.1016/j.ejphar.2009.10.011

7. ScienceDaily. (2018, April 10). *Does physical activity influence the health of future offspring?* ScienceDaily. https://www.sciencedaily.com/releases/2018/04/180410132900.htm.

8. Alegría-Torres JA, Baccarelli A, Bollati V. Epigenetics and lifestyle. Epigenomics. 2011 Jun;3(3):267-77. doi: 10.2217/epi.11.22. PMID: 22122337; PMCID: PMC3752894.

4. Behavioral Neuroscience:

1. *Sleep and Obesity.* Obesity Prevention Source. (2016, April 13). https://www.hsph.harvard.edu/obesity-prevention-source/obesity-causes/sleep-and-obesity/.

2. *The study illuminates the 'pain' of social rejection*—University of Michigan News. (2011, March 25). https://news.umich.edu/study-illuminates-the-pain-of-social-rejection/.

3. Woods, C., Mutrie, N., & Scott, M. (2002). Physical activity intervention: A Transtheoretical Model-based Intervention designed to help sedentary young adults become active. *Health Education Research, 17*(4), 451–460. https://doi.org/10.1093/her.17.4.451

4. Boston University School of Public Health. (n.d.). *The Social Cognitive Theory*. Behavioral Change Models. https://sphweb.bumc.bu.edu/otlt/MPH-Modules/SB/BehavioralChangeTheories/BehavioralChangeTheories5.html.

5. Bandura, Albert (2010), "Self-Efficacy," *The Corsini Encyclopedia of Psychology*, American Cancer Society, pp. 1–3, doi:10.1002/9780470479216.corpsy0836, ISBN 978-0-470-47921-6, retrieved 2021-03-20

6. Vahidi, S. (2015, June 16). *What influences SELF-EFFICACY?* The National Research Center on the Gifted and Talented 1990-2013. https://nrcgt.uconn.edu/underachievement_study/self-efficacy/se_section2/.

7. Ashford S, Edmunds J, French DP. What is the best way to change self-efficacy to promote lifestyle and recreational physical activity? A systematic review with meta-analysis. Br J Health Psychol. 2010 May;15(Pt 2):265-88. doi: 10.1348/135910709X461752. Epub 2009 Jul 7. PMID: 19586583.

8. Rosenstock, I. M. (1974). The health belief model and preventive health behavior. *Health Education Monographs*, *2*(4), 354–386. https://doi.org/10.1177/109019817400200405

9. Janz, N. K., & Becker, H. M. (1984). The health belief model: A decade later. Health Education Quarterly, 11, 1–47.

10. Fishbein, M., & Ajzen, I. (1975). *Belief, Attitude, Intention, and Behavior: An Introduction to Theory and Research*. Reading, MA: Addison-Wesley.

11. Ryan, R., & Deci, E. (2000). Self-determination theory and the facilitation of intrinsic motivation, social development, and well-being. *American Psychologist*, *55*(1), 68–78. https://doi.org/10.1037/0003-066x.55.1.68

12. Kahneman, D. (1999). Objective happiness. In D. Kahneman, E. Diener, & N. Schwarz (Eds.), Wellbeing: The foundations of hedonic psychology (pp. 3–25). New York: Russell Sage Foundation.

5. Retrain Your Brain

1. Brown, Daphne. Negative Experiences in Physical Education Class and Avoidance of Exercise. *FHSU scholars - fort hays state university*. (n.d.). Retrieved June 22, 2022, from https://scholars.fhsu.edu/cgi/viewcontent.cgi?article=1054&context=theses

2. Berg, S. (2021, November 19). *What doctors wish patients knew about decision fatigue*. American Medical Association. Retrieved June 22, 2022, from https://www.ama-assn.org/delivering-care/public-health/what-doctors-wish-patients-knew-about-decision-fatigue#:~:text=Decision%20fatigue%20is%20%E2%80%9Cthe%20idea,more%20difficult%20it%20can%20become.%E2%80%9D

3. Hamasaki, H. (2020). Effects of diaphragmatic breathing on Health: A Narrative Review. *Medicines*, *7*(10), 65. https://doi.org/10.3390/medicines7100065

4. Mayo Foundation for Medical Education and Research. (2022, April 29). *A beginner's guide to meditation*. Mayo Clinic. Retrieved June 22, 2022, from https://www.mayoclinic.org/tests-procedures/meditation/in-depth/meditation/art-20045858

6. Age and Longevity: How Epigenetics

1. World Health Organization. (n.d.). *Decade of Healthy Ageing (2021-2030)*. World Health Organization. Retrieved January 21, 2022, from https://www.who.int/initiatives/decade-of-healthy-ageing

2. Taylor, M. (2019, April 22). *A 'fountain of youth' pill? Sure, if you're a mouse.* Kaiser Health News. Retrieved January 21, 2022, from https://khn.org/news/a-fountain-of-youth-pill-sure-if-youre-a-mouse/

3. Sinclair, D., & LaPlante, M. D. (2021). *Lifespan: Why we age and why we don't have to.* Harper Thorsons.

4. Willcox DC; Willcox BJ; Shimajiri S;Kurechi S;Suzuki M; (n.d.). *Aging gracefully: A retrospective analysis of functional status in Okinawan centenarians.* The American journal of geriatric psychiatry: official journal of the American Association for Geriatric Psychiatry. Retrieved June 22, 2022, from https://pubmed.ncbi.nlm.nih.gov/17322136/

5. *Blue zones-live longer, better 2021 - blue zones.* Blue Zones - Live Better, Longer. (2022, June 21). Retrieved June 22, 2022, from https://www.bluezones.com/

7. How to Stick to a Difficult Regimen

1. Horan, R. D., Bulte, E., & Shogren, J. F. (2005). How trade saved humanity from biological exclusion: An economic theory of neanderthal extinction. *Journal of Economic Behavior & Organization, 58*(1), 1–29. https://doi.org/10.1016/j.jebo.2004.03.009

8. Hormones and You

1. *The Nobel Prize: Women who changed science: Elizabeth Blackburn.* The official website of the Nobel Prize - NobelPrize.org. (n.d.). Retrieved June 22, 2022, from https://www.nobelprize.org/womenwhochangedscience/stories/elizabeth-blackburn

2. Blackburn, E. H., & Epel, E. (2018). *The telomere effect: A revolutionary approach to living younger, healthier, longer.* Orion Spring.

3. Weintraub, K. (2017, January 4). *How to control aging.* Scientific American. Retrieved June 22, 2022, from https://www.scientificamerican.com/article/how-to-control-aging/

4. Fung, J. (2016). *The obesity code: Unlocking the secrets of Weight Loss.* Greystone Books.

5. E. on J. (2020, March 6). *Insulin resistance occurs when insulin levels are sufficiently high over a prolonged period of time causing the body's own sensitivity to the hormone to be reduced.* Diabetes. Retrieved June 22, 2022, from https://www.diabetes.co.uk/insulin-resistance.html

6. Mayo Foundation for Medical Education and Research. (2021, July 8). *Chronic stress puts your health at risk.* Mayo Clinic. Retrieved June 22, 2022, from https://www.mayoclinic.org/healthy-lifestyle/stress-management/in-depth/stress/art-20046037#:~:text=Cortisol%2C%20the%20primary%20stress%20hormone,fight%2Dor%2Dflight%20situation.

7. Sleep loss results in an elevation of cortisol levels the next evening. (1997). *Sleep.* https://doi.org/10.1093/sleep/20.10.865

8. Horng, H.-C., Chang, W.-H., Yeh, C.-C., Huang, B.-S., Chang, C.-P., Chen, Y.-J., Tsui, K.-H., & Wang, P.-H. (2017). Estrogen effects on wound healing. *International Journal of Molecular Sciences, 18*(11), 2325. https://doi.org/10.3390/ijms18112325

9. Cagnacci, A., & Venier, M. (2019). The controversial history of Hormone Replacement therapy. *Medicina, 55*(9), 602. https://doi.org/10.3390/medicina55090602

10. MediLexicon International. (n.d.). *Phytoestrogens: Benefits, risks, and food list*. Medical News Today. Retrieved June 22, 2022, from https://www.medicalnewstoday.com/arti cles/320630#how-they-work

11. Reed, K. E., Camargo, J., Hamilton-Reeves, J., Kurzer, M., & Messina, M. (2021). Neither soy nor isoflavone intake affects male reproductive hormones: An expanded and updated meta-analysis of Clinical Studies. *Reproductive Toxicology, 100*, 60–67. https://doi.org/10.1016/j.reprotox.2020.12.019

12. Ramasamy, R., Osterberg, E. C., & Bernie, A. M. (2014). Risks of testosterone replace-ment therapy in men. *Indian Journal of Urology, 30*(1), 2. https://doi.org/10.4103/0970-1591.124197

13. Afrisham, R., Sadegh-Nejadi, S., Soliemani Far, O., Kooti, W., Ashtary-Larky, D., Alamiri, F., Aberomand, M., Najjar-Asl, S., & Khaneh-Keshi, A. (2016). Salivary testosterone levels under psychological stress and its relationship with rumination and five personality traits in medical students. *Psychiatry Investigation, 13*(6), 637. https://doi.org/10.4306/pi.2016.13.6.637

14. Seithikurippu R, A. M. (2015). Melatonin, the hormone of darkness: From sleep promotion to ebola treatment. *Brain Disorders & Therapy, 04*(01). https://doi.org/10.4172/2168-975x.1000151

15. Reiter, R. J., Mayo, J. C., Tan, D.-X., Sainz, R. M., Alatorre-Jimenez, M., & Qin, L. (2016). Melatonin as an antioxidant: Under promises but over delivers. *Journal of Pineal Research, 61*(3), 253–278. https://doi.org/10.1111/jpi.12360

16. Mayo Foundation for Medical Education and Research. (2021, November 13). *Human growth hormone (HGH): Does it slow aging?* Mayo Clinic. Retrieved June 22, 2022, from https://www.mayoclinic.org/healthy-lifestyle/healthy-aging/in-depth/growth-hormone/art-20045735#:~:text=Growth%20hormone%20fuels%20child hood%20growth,of%20growth%20hormone%20it%20produces.

17. Cronkleton, E. (2019, March 29). *HGH: Side effects in men and women*. Healthline. Retrieved June 27, 2022, from https://www.healthline.com/health/hgh-side-effects#side-effects

18. Sattler, F. R. (2013). Growth hormone in the aging male. *Best Practice & Research Clinical Endocrinology & Metabolism, 27*(4), 541–555. https://doi.org/10.1016/j.beem.2013.05.003

10. Muscle Mass: Your Secret Ally in Weight Loss

1. Yeung, S. S. Y., Reijnierse, E. M., Pham, V. K., Trappenburg, M. C., Lim, W. K., Meskers, C. G. M., & Maier, A. B. (2019). Sarcopenia and its association with falls and fractures in older adults: A systematic review and meta-analysis. *Journal of Cachexia, Sarcopenia and Muscle, 10*(3), 485–500. https://doi.org/10.1002/jcsm.12411

2. Morris, R., & O'Riordan, S. (2017). Prevention of falls in hospital. *Clinical Medicine, 17*(4), 360–362. https://doi.org/10.7861/clinmedicine.17-4-360

3. Cruz-Jentoft, A. J. (2018). Sarcopenia: Preventable and reversible. *Practical Issues in Geriatrics*, 47–52. https://doi.org/10.1007/978-3-319-96529-1_5

4. Moore, L. M. |. (2009, June 8). *Liam Hoekstra, the 'world strongest toddler' to hit TV*. mlive. Retrieved June 27, 2022, from https://www.mlive.com/news/muskegon/2009/06/liam_hoekstra_the_world_strong.html#:~:text=The%20only%20other%20com pany%20that,meals%20and%20snacks%20a%20day.

5. Walston, J. D. (2012). Sarcopenia in older adults. *Current Opinion in Rheumatology*, *24*(6), 623–627. https://doi.org/10.1097/bor.0b013e328358d59b
6. Haase, C. B., Brodersen, J. B., & Bülow, J. (2022). Sarcopenia: Early prevention or overdiagnosis? *BMJ*. https://doi.org/10.1136/bmj-2019-052592

11. Health & Fitness Hacks: Vibration Technology

1. Marin, P. and Rhea, M. (2010). Effects Of Vibration Training on Muscle Strength: A meta-Analysis, The Journal of Strength & Conditioning 24(2), 548-556.
2. Cristi-Montero, C., Cuevas, M.J., & Collado, P. S. Whole-body Vibration Training as A complement to Programs Aimed at Weight Loss. Nutr Hosp. 2013;28(5):1365-1371.
3. Marin, P. and Rhea, M. (2010). Effects Of Vibration Training on Muscle Strength: A A meta-Analysis, Journal of Strength & Conditioning 24(2), 548-556.
4. Zago, M., Capodaglio, P., Ferrario, C., Tarabini, M., & Galli, M. (2018). Whole-body vibration training in obese subjects: A systematic review. PLOS One 13(9), 1-20.
5. Ibid

12. The Truth About Weight Loss

1. Benton, D., & Young, H. A. (2017). Reducing calorie intake may not help you lose body weight. *Perspectives on Psychological Science*, *12*(5), 703–714. https://doi.org/10.1177/1745691617690878
2. Pontzer, H. (2021). *Burn: New research blows the lid off how we really burn calories, lose weight, and stay healthy*. Avery, an imprint of Penguin Random House.
3. *Ibid*
4. Sinclair, D., & LaPlante, M. D. (2021). *Lifespan: Why we age and why we don't have to*. Harper Thorsons.
5. Pontzer, H. (2021). *Burn: New research blows the lid off how we really burn calories, lose weight, and stay healthy*. Avery, an imprint of Penguin Random House.
6. Pontzer, H. (2021). *Burn: New research blows the lid off how we really burn calories, lose weight, and stay healthy*. Avery, an imprint of Penguin Random House.
7. Fung, J. (2016). *The obesity code: Unlocking the secrets of Weight Loss.*
8. Pontzer, H. (2021). *Burn: New research blows the lid off how we really burn calories, lose weight, and stay healthy*. Avery, an imprint of Penguin Random House.
9. *Plant-based fats: Better for the heart than animal fats?* Harvard Health. (2018, June 1). Retrieved July 1, 2022, from https://www.health.harvard.edu/heart-health/plant-based-fats-better-for-the-heart-than-animal-fats#:~:text=Heart%20disease%20risk%20was%20lower,of%20dying%20from%20any%20cause.

13. The Truth About Exercise

1. Pontzer, H. (2021). *Burn: New research blows the lid off how we really burn calories, lose weight, and stay healthy*. Avery, an imprint of Penguin Random House.

2. Lindell, J. (2019, November 22). *How fast does a cheetah run?* Sciencing. Retrieved July 1, 2022, from https://sciencing.com/how-fast-does-cheetah-run-4577113.html

3. Rosati, A. (2018, February 26). *Food for thought: Was cooking a pivotal step in human evolution?* Scientific American. Retrieved July 1, 2022, from https://www.scientificamerican.com/article/food-for-thought-was-cooking-a-pivotal-step-in-human-evolution/

4. Sinclair, D., & LaPlante, M. D. (2021). *Lifespan: Why we age and why we don't have to.* Harper Thorsons.

5. Pontzer, H. (2021). *Burn: New research blows the lid off how we really burn calories, lose weight, and stay healthy.* Avery, an imprint of Penguin Random House.

6. Sinclair, D., & LaPlante, M. D. (2021). *Lifespan: Why we age and why we don't have to.* Harper Thorsons.

7. Buyken, A. E., Flood, V., Empson, M., Rochtchina, E., Barclay, A. W., Brand-Miller, J., & Mitchell, P. (2010). Carbohydrate nutrition and inflammatory disease mortality in older adults. *The American Journal of Clinical Nutrition, 92*(3), 634–643. https://doi.org/10.3945/ajcn.2010.29390

8. Zheng, G., Qiu, P., Xia, R., Lin, H., Ye, B., Tao, J., & Chen, L. (2019). Effect of aerobic exercise on inflammatory markers in healthy middle-aged and older adults: A systematic review and meta-analysis of randomized controlled trials. *Frontiers in Aging Neuroscience, 11*. https://doi.org/10.3389/fnagi.2019.00098

9. Meydani, S. N., Das, S. K., Pieper, C. F., Lewis, M. R., Klein, S., Dixit, V. D., Gupta, A. K., Villareal, D. T., Bhapkar, M., Huang, M., Fuss, P. J., Roberts, S. B., Holloszy, J. O., & Fontana, L. (2016). Long-term moderate calorie restriction inhibits inflammation without impairing cell-mediated immunity: A randomized controlled trial in non-obese humans. *Aging, 8*(7), 1416–1431. https://doi.org/10.18632/aging.100994

14. The Spirituality of Health and Weight Loss

1. Crossway. (2019). *Esv new christian's Bible: English standard version containing the old and new testaments, personal reference bible.*

2. Harris, J. C. (2014). Anorexia nervosa and anorexia mirabilis. *JAMA Psychiatry, 71*(11), 1212. https://doi.org/10.1001/jamapsychiatry.2013.2765

Printed in Great Britain
by Amazon

23170008R00106